Stem Cell Research in Lab Animals

NIPA® GENX ELECTRONIC RESOURCES & SOLUTIONS P. LTD.
New Delhi-110 034

Stem Cell Research in Lab Animals

Swapan Kumar Maiti
Principal Scientist
Division of Surgery
ICAR-Indian Veterinary Research Institute
Izatnagar, Uttar Pradesh, India

NIPA® GENX ELECTRONIC RESOURCES & SOLUTIONS P. LTD.
New Delhi-110 034

NIPA® GENX ELECTRONIC RESOURCES & SOLUTIONS P. LTD.

101,103, Vikas Surya Plaza, CU Block
L.S.C. Market, Pitam Pura, New Delhi-110 034
Ph : +91 11 27341616, 27341717, 27341718
E-mail: newindiapublishingagency@gmail.com
web: www.nipabooks.com

For customer assistance, please contact
Phone: + 91-11-27 34 17 17
Fax: + 91-11- 27 34 16 16
E-Mail: feedbacks@nipabooks.com

ISBN: 978-93-58870-20-6

Composed and Designed by NIPA®.

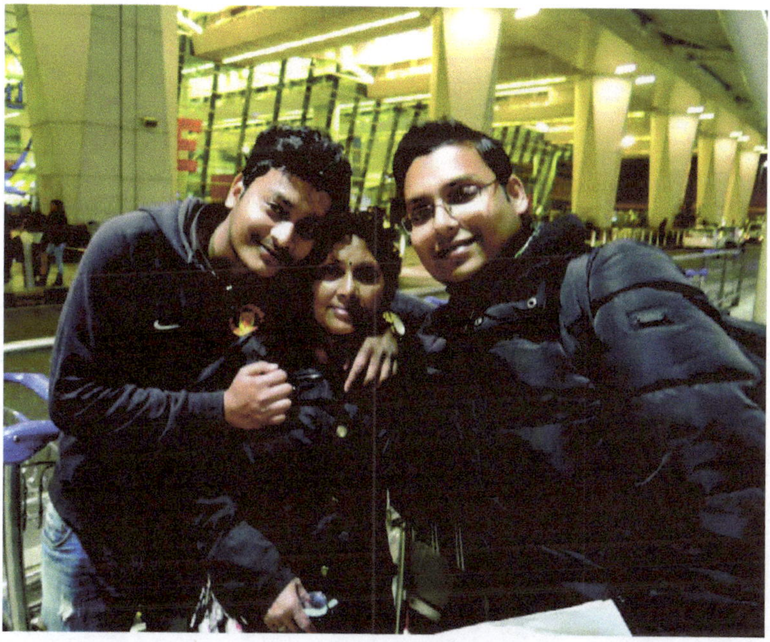

Dedicated to

My Beloved Family

Acknowledgement

I am grateful to the Director and Joint Directors of Indian Veterinary Research Institute, Izatnagar (UP) for their generous help and support towards this publication. I wish to acknowledge the authors and publishers of different reference books/papers consulted for the preparation of this task with special mention to "Stem Cells from Bench to Beside" (Bongso and Lee, Eds, World Scientific Publishing Company); "Essential of Stem Cell Biology" (Robert Lanza, Ed, Elsevier Academic Press), and "Stem Cell Research: Medical Applications & Ethical Controversy" (Joseph Panno, Ed) for stem cell introduction, definition and application.

Help and wholehearted support extended by all the faculty members in general, especially Dr Naveen Kumar, Principal Scientist and my beloved PG students of Surgery Division, IVRI especially Drs Bhagyashree K Bhadane, Ninu A R, Shiva Kumar M U, Sandeep Kumar, Tamil Mahan, Sangeetha P, Divya Mohan Shivaraju S and Kalaiselvan E in particular to bring out the publication are duly acknowledged. I have no hesitation to acknowledge their hard research work which is the backbone of this book; actually they are the co-authors of this book.

I gratefully acknowledge to Department of Biotechnology (DBT) for providing necessary funds and facility to author for carry out stem cell research under approved research project as Principal Investigator and also duly acknowledge their manual on "Guidelines for Stem Cell Research and Therapy"-from which some definitions have been reproduce in this book.

Special thanks and acknowledgements are also due to Mr Bob Harman, CEO, Vet Stem Biopharma Inc, USA for giving permission to reproduce one figure and some text in this book.

Mere coining of words is not enough for encompassing the whole hearted support and sacrifice of my beloved wife Rina and sons-Akashneel and Abhinandan who gave me all the strength and courage to accomplish this arduous task.

I would appreciate to receive any suggestion and constructive criticism about the publication and my efforts would be to further improve more subject and latest information in the next edition. Hope my efforts will help to the clinicians researchers and students to alleviates the suffering of animal pain through stem cell technology.

Date: 6th August, 2019 **Swapan Kumar Maiti**

Preface

This book covers most of the topics with latest information on stem cell in general and mesenchymal stem cell (MSC) research in particular. The book is divided into 17 chapters covering almost all aspect of stem cell technology including definition of different types of stem cells, isolation of MSC from different animals, culture and characteristics of mesenchymal stem cell, osteoinduction potential of MSC, protocol for isolation of bone marrow derived MSC, fat derived MSC, embryonic stem cells (ESC), protocol for MSC passaging. This book also includes different research findings on application of bioengineered stem cell technologies in skin wound healing, burn wound healing, critical bone defect healing, large bone defect healing, corneal wound healing and in liver regeneration. The main objective of this book is to provide the latest information to meet the requirements of not only undergraduate and post graduates research scholars but also to the teachers, biologists and clinician involved in animal treatment and research. The book contains more than 150 good quality colour photographs of stem cell isolation, stem cell culture, stem cell morphology, stem cell characteristics and stem cell application in different surgical interventions.

This book would be of immense use to the students, teachers and research scholars engaged in the filed of stem cell technology.

Author

Contents

1

Stem Cells: Definition and Its Application

Stem cell research is one of the most important and promising areas of research in biological science in recent times. The stem cell technology has revolutionized modern biology. It is playing a major role for improving human as well as animal health by controlling number of incurable degenerative diseases and restoration of damage to organs via transplantation therapy. Stem cells are a specific group of cells that remain in an undifferentiated state and can be found in embryos, fetuses and adult individuals. Stem cells are primitive, undifferentiated cells present in almost every tissue that have the ability to differentiate into different types of tissue like bone, tendon, ligament, cartilage etc. Bone marrow stem cell is the ideal stem cell that is unspecialized and can undergo lineage specific differentiation into bone or blood cells under different signals or environment with new special function. Several verities of stem cells have been isolated and identified *in vivo* and *in vitro*. The two broad types of mammalian stem cells are embryonic stem cells that are found in blastocyst, and adult stem cells that are found in adult tissue, bone marrow.

The stem cells are nature's miracle. Stem cells are unspecialized cells and retain the ability to renew them through mitotic cell division and can differentiate into a diverse range of specialized cell types. Stem cells have the following abilities: proliferate and self-renew for a number of generations; differentiate into the major lineages of the tissue they are derived from and regenerate the tissue and/or organ they are derived form. Stem cells are defined classically by the following these criteria. First, self-renewal: stem cells undergo self-renewing cell divisions; that is, they can give rise to at least one daughter cell that is identical to the initial cell; the ability to go through many cycles of cell division (mitosis) while maintaining the undifferentiated state. This property is essential to maintain the stem cell pool. Second, potency: the capacity to differentiate into specialized cell types. Stem cells undergo lineage commitment and differentiation, giving rise to more differentiated progenitors, precursor cells, and ultimately terminally differentiated cells. This requires stem cells to either totipotent, pluripotent or multipotent- to give rise to any mature cell type. Third, stem cells repopulate in a robust fashion, a given tissue where they differentiate in response to specific cause to differentiate into cell types of that tissue which can take over the function of that tissue (Verfaillie, 2006). If all these criteria can be met from a cell within a population then, it can be defined as a stem cell.

Definition

Stem cells: Cells capable of self-replication, proliferation and differentiation.

Adult stem cell: A stem cell derived from the tissues or organs of an organism after birth. Adult stem cells, also known as somatic stem cells: cells which maintain and repair the tissue in which they are found. They can be found in children, as well as adults.

Embryonic stem cell: Stem cells are derived from the inner cell mass up to the stage of blastocyst. These cells can be cultured indefinitely under *in vitro* conditions that allow proliferation without differentiation, but have the potential of differentiating into any cell of the body.

Cord blood stem cells: Stem cells are collected from the umbilical cord at birth that can produce all of the blood cells in the body (hematopoietic).

Fetal stem cell: A stem cell derived from fetal tissue, including placenta. A distinction is drawn between the fetal germ cells, from which the gametes develop, and the fetal somatic cell, from which rest of the organism develops.

Mesenchymal stem cells: Stem cells present in human bone marrow and umbilical cord that have been shown to differentiate into a variety of cell types.

Totipotent stem cell (Omnipotent): Able to give rise to all cell types, including cells of the trophoectoderm lineage. Example: fertilized egg, morula. Stem cells can differentiate into embryonic and extra embryonic cells and these cells can construct a complete and viable organism. At two to three days after fertilization, an embryo consists of identical cells (morula), which are totipotent. They are totally unspecialized and have the capacity to differentiate into any of the cells, which will constitute the fetus and the placenta and membranes around the fetus.

Pluripotent stem cell: Able to give rise to differentiated cells of all three germ layers (mesoderm, endoderm and ectoderm), in other words- cells derived from any of the three germ layers. Pluripotent stem cells are the descendants of totipotent cells. Cells of the inner cell mass of blastocyst and ES cells are pluripotent. Pluripotent stem cell has the potential to generate into every cell type in the body, but cannot develop into an embryo on its own. The most well-known type of pluripotent stem cell is the embryonic stem cell. However, since the generation of embryonic stem cells involves destruction of embryo, there has been much controversy surrounding their use. Further, because embryonic stem cells can only be derived from embryos, it has so far not been feasible to create patient-matched embryonic stem cell lines.

Multipotent stem cell: Stem cells are those which are capable of giving rise to several different types of specialized cells constituting a specific tissue or organ. Multipotent stem cells can differentiate into a number of cell types, but produce only cells of a closely related family of cells, eg, hematopoietic stem cells differentiate into red blood cells, white blood cells, platelets, etc.; bone marrow derived stem cells differentiate into osteogenic, chondrogenic or adipogenic cells.

Oligopotent stem cells: Stem cell can differentiate into only a few cell types, such as lymphoid or myeloid stem cells

Unipotent stem cell: Stem cells can differentiate only one cell type, their own, but have the property of self-renewal which distinguishes them non-stem cell (progenitor cells- cannot self renewal) (e.g. muscle stem cells)

Induced pluripotent stem cells (iPS cells): A type of pluripotent stem cell that can be generated directly from adult cells. The iPSC technology was pioneered by Shinya Yamanaka's lab in Kyoto, Japan, who showed in 2006 that the introduction of four specific genes encoding transcription factors could convert adult cells into pluripotent stem cells. He was awarded the 2012 Nobel Prize along with Sir John Gurdon "for the discovery that mature cells can be reprogrammed to become pluripotent."

Parthenogenetic stem cell: Stem cells derived from an egg that undergone a process known as parthenogenesis. Parthenogenesis is the biological phenomenon by which an egg can develop into an embryo in the absence of sperm. Therefore, sometimes it is also called as a "Virgin birth" in which an embryo is created from solely from a female oocyte without any genetic contribution from a male. In animals, parthenogenesis means development of an embryo from an unfertilized egg cell. It has been reported in about 70 lower species of invertebrates. Flies, ants, lizards, snakes, fish, birds, amphibians, honeybees are routinely reproduce in this manner.

Cell line: Cells of common descent continuously cultured in the laboratory is referred to as a cell line

Somatic stem cells: An undifferentiated cell found among differentiated cells in a tissue or organ, which can renew itself and can differentiate to yield the major specialized cell types of the tissue or organ.

Stem cell bank: A facility that is responsible for accessioning, processing, packaging, labeling, storage and delivery of a finished stem cell line issued under its name. It is required to characterize the cells, provide quality assurance and meet the laid down standards and procedure.

Chimera: An animal composed of cells originating from two or more embryos produced. For example, by injecting embryonic stem cells into a blastocyst of different genotype.

Stem cell plasticity: Apparent ability of a stem cell/ progenitor cell fated to a given tissue to acquire a differentiated phenotype of a different tissue.

Niche: The local microenvironment that support stem cell maintenance and self-renewal.

Feeder layer: Cells used in co-culture to maintain pluripotent nature of stem cells.

Multipotent Mesenchymal Stromal cells (MSC): Bone marrow, in addition to hematopoietic stem cells (HSC) also contains stromal stem cells, referred to as MSCs. Mesenchymal stem cells (MSCs), also termed multipotent mesenchymal stromal cells, are a phenotypically and functionally heterogeneous cell population. In culture, they are defined as plastic-adherent, fibroblast-like cells which are able to self-renew and differentiate into bone, adipose and cartilage tissue. MSCs are first described by Friedenstein and colleagues in 1974 as cells capable of giving rise to fibroblast-like colonies that could differentiate into osteocytes, chondrocytes and adipocytes. Owen and Friedenstein (1988) called this cell an osteogenic stem cell or a BM stromal cell. Although the pioneering work of Friedenstein is firmly established, the concept of non-hematopoietic stem cell comes into light only after the publication of similar work by Pittenger *et al.* (1999). The term mesenchymal stem cells (MSCs) are first coined by Caplan (1991) as an alternative to "stromal" or "osteogenic" stem cell.

Sources: Generally isolated from bone marrow, but they are also isolated from a variety of tissues including umbilical cord blood, chorionic villi of the placenta, Wharton's jelly, peripheral blood, fetal liver and lung, adipose tissue, skeletal muscle, periosteum, deciduous teeth, amniotic fluid, synovium and the circulatory system. Bone marrow and periosteum sources are richest in young animals with their numbers diminishing, but still present in old age. MSC numbers and biologic activity are greatest in metaphyseal bone and areas of thick and vascular periosteum.

Reported Frequency of MSC isolated from different sources

- Bone Marrow: 1 in 10^5
- Adipose tissue : 2 in 100
- Cord Blood: 0-2 in 500
- Wharton's Jelly :1 in 333

Morphology

Mesenchymal stem cells are characterized morphologically by a small cell body with a few cell processes that are long and thin. The cell body contains a large, round nucleus with a prominent nucleolus which is surrounded by finely dispersed chromatin particles, giving the nucleus a clear appearance. The remainder of the cell body contains a small amount of Golgi apparatus, rough endoplasmic reticulum, mitochondria, and polyribosome. The cells, which are long and thin, are widely dispersed and the adjacent extracellular matrix is populated by a few reticular fibrils but is devoid of the other types of collagen fibrils (MSC Wikipedia).

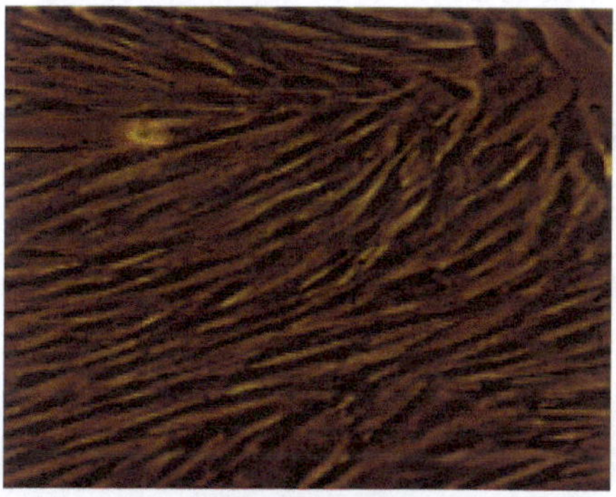

Equine MSC

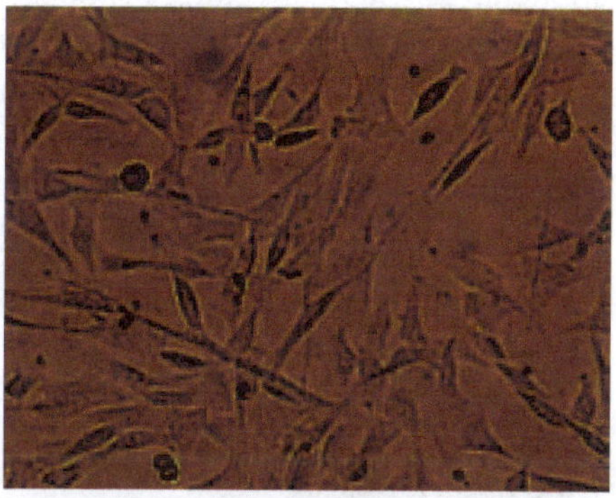

Canine MSC

MSC Phenotype

MSC identification relies on a combination of positively and negatively expressed markers that facilitates their characterization among other cellular subsets . A recent publication from the International Society for Cellular Therapy has come out with three minimal criteria for defining human 'multipotent mesenchymal stromal cells' (MSC). First, MSC must be plastic adherent when maintained in standard culture conditions. Second, MSC must express CD105, CD73, and CD90, and lack CD45, CD34, CD14 (or CD11b), CD79a (or CD19) and HLA DR surface molecules. Lastly, MSC must differentiate to osteoblasts, adipocytes and chondroblasts *in vitro* (Dominici *et al*., 2006).

Differentiation of MSC

MSCs are multipotential cells capable of differentiating into osteoblasts (bone), chondrocytes (cartilage), adipocytes (adipose tissue), tenocytes (tendon), skeletal muscle, cardiac muscle, neural cells and connective tissues. There is some recent evidence that there is a rare cell within MSC cultures that is pluripotent and can give rise not only to mesodermal but to endodermal tissues. The authors have called this a Multipotent Adult Progenitor Cell.

Isolation of MSC

Isolation techniques generally are based on the adherent properties of the MSC. Density gradient centrifugation is employed initially to separate nucleated MSC. As the cells are cultured, MSC adhere to the flask surface. The non-adherent cells are removed with the culture medium when it is changed, concentrating the MSC. The cells are repeatedly passage, expanding the cell population, until a pure culture is produced.

MSCs comprise a mere 0.01-0.0001% of total bone marrow nucleated cells and need *in vitro* cell culture expansion in order to get sufficient numbers for clinical applications. Standard culture expansion protocols for MSCs involve attachment of the cells to the plastic surface of a culture flask. The attached cells following an initial lag phase expand through rapid divisions and turn confluent before they enter into stationary phase. Morphologically they are spindle shaped and resemble fibroblast culture, but when confluent they acquire a flattened morphology. MSC culture media comprises a basal medium, qualified fetal calf serum, and different growth factors and hormones like TGF β, hydrocortisone and FGF 2. MSC culture was first established by Friedenstein and his colleagues by virtue of the physical propensity of MSCs to adhere to plastic flasks.

Characteristics of MSC

1. **Immunomodulation**: MSC exhibit immunomodulatory properties through the release of bioactive agents such as cytokines that can inhibit autoimmune response. In general, *in vitro* studies demonstrate those bone marrow-derived MSCs (BM-MSCs) and adipose –derived MSC (AD-MSCs) limit inflammatory responses and promote anti-inflammatory pathways. When present in an inflammatory environment, data demonstrate that BM-MSCs may alter the cytokine secretion profile of dendritic cell (DC) subsets and T-cell subsets causing a shift from a pro-inflammatory environment to an anti- inflammatory to tolerant environment. BM-MSCs do not express MHC class II antigens or costimulatory molecules and they suppress T cell proliferation. AD-MSC suppress mixed lymphocyte reactions and inhibits T cell proliferation

induced by a third cell type or by mitogenic factors. Both BM-MSC and AD-MSC are able to control lethal graft versus host diseases (GVHD) in mice after haploidentical hematopoietic transplantation.

2. **Trophic Support**: Multiple studies demonstrate that MSCs secrete bioactive levels of cytokines and growth factors that support angiogenesis, tissue remodeling, differentiation and anti-apoptotic events such as vascular endothelial growth factor (VEGF), hepatocyte growth factor (HGF), basic fibroblast growth factor (bFGF) and transforming growth factor- β (TGF-β).

3. **Differentiation:** BM-MSCs and adipose derived MSC demonstrate a diverse plasticity, including differentiation into adipo-, osteo-, chondro-, myo-, cardiomyo-, endothelial, hepato-, neuro-, epithelial and hematopoietic lineages. These data supported by *in vivo* experiments and functional studies that demonstrate the regenerative capacity of adipose-derived MSC and BM-MSC to repair damaged or diseased tissue via transplant engraftment and differentiation.

4. **Homing**: Homing (chemotaxis) is an event by which a cell migrates from one area of the body to a distant site where it may be needed for a given physiological event. Homing is an important function of MSCs and other progenitor cells and one mechanism by which intravenous or parenteral administration of MSCs permits an auto-transplanted therapeutic cell to effectively target a specific area of pathology. It has been demonstrated that labeled cells of bone lineage injected intravenously into mice can engraft, form bone and give rise to osteocytes and bone lining cells detectable on the mouse femur.

5. **Revascularization**: BM-MSCs and adipose derived MSC contain endothelial progenitor cells that assist in angiogenesis and neovascularization by the secretion of cytokines, such as hepatic growth factor (HGF), vascular endothelial growth factor (VEGF), placental growth factor (PGF), transforming growth factor (TGF- β), fibroblast growth factor (FGF) and angiopoietin. It has been examined the effect of intravenous administration of BM-MSCs after cerebral arterial occlusion in the rat and demonstrated new capillary formation, increased vessel formation and increased VEGF expression in the areas of the lesion. In an *in vivo* model of hind limb ischemia, intravenous injection of AD-MSC are associated with an increase in blood flow and capillary density and incorporation of the cells in the leg vasculature. It is reported that nude mice with ischemic hind limbs demonstrate marked perfusion improvement when treated with human AD-MSC.

6. **Anti-apoptosis**: Apoptosis is defined s a programmed cell death or "cell suicide", an event that is genetically controlled. Under normal conditions, apoptosis determines the lifespan and coordinated removal of cells. Unlike necrosis, apoptosis cells are typically intact during their removal (phagocytosis). Different workers demonstrate this effect in actually injured tissue denied critical blood-flow resulting in ischemia. AD-MSC significantly reduce endothelial cell apoptosis. It has been also demonstrated that BM-MSCs express factors that support cell survival and avoid apoptosis thereby preserving cells that would otherwise be destroyed (Vet Stem Biopharma website).
7. **Neuroprotection**: MSC can promote neuroprotection in the CNS of patients with MSC which may prevent the progression of the disease to chronic disability. The mechanism includes inhibiting apoptosis which will prevent the death of healthy cells and prevent gliosis which will prevent the formation of glial scar.
8. **Neuroregeneration**: MSC have the ability to stimulate neuroregeneration by contributing to cell replacement through differentiating into neural stem cells in response to inflammation. The neural stem cells can then promote the repair of damaged axons of nerve tissue (MSC Wikipedia)

Therapeutic application of mesenchymal stem cells

Mesenchymal stem cells have generated a great amount of enthusiasm as a novel therapeutic tool for a variety of incurable degenerative and inflammatory disease. Mesenchymal stem cells (MSCs) are multipotent stem cells and ability to self-renewal and can differentiate into several mesodermal cell types including osteoblasts, chondrocytes, adipocytes, myocytes, tenocytes, beta-pancreatic islets cells and neuronal cells. MSCs are now immense therapeutic interest because they have potentiality to treat a wide range of acute degenerative and inflammatory diseases. MSCs are advantageous over other stem cells like ES for many reasons. First, they avoid the ethical controversy and teratoma formation that surround embryonic stem cell research. Second, many studies confirm that MSCs are immune-privileged, and therefore, represent an advantageous cell type for allogenic transplantation, reducing the risks of rejection and complications of cell transplantation therapy.

Mesenchymal stem cells uses in clinical regenerative medicine owing to their unique immunomodulatory and engraftment promoting properties. The mechanisms through which MSC exert their therapeutic potential rely on some very important biological properties of these cells: the ability to secrete some soluble molecules capable of stimulating survival and recovery of injured cells (trophic support); the ability to home to sites of inflammation following tissue injury when injected parenteral (homing); the ability to differentiate into various cell types (differentiation) and lack of immunogenicity and the ability to perform immunomodulatory function.

Some striking examples of the therapeutic uses of MSCs have been reported recently in applications such as coronary artery disease, cardio-vascular repair, spinal cord injury, Parkinson's disease, liver regeneration, diabetes and leukemia. In orthopedics, stem cell therapy is now routinely uses in bone, cartilage and tendon repair and in the treatment of osteoarthritis.

These cells have been successfully employed in graft versus host disease treatment, heart regeneration after infarct, cartilage and bone repair, skin wounds healing, neuronal regeneration and many others. The list of reports indicating that MSCs contribute to tissue repair in vivo enlarges. There are examples of MSC utilization in the repair of kidney, muscle and lung. The cells are also found to promote angiogenesis. Of special importance is their use in the treatment of osteogenesis imperfecta, which appeared to be the only reasonable therapeutic strategy. MSCs seem to represent a future powerful tool in regenerative medicine (Bobis *et al.*, 2006).

1. **Tendon repair**- Significant improvements using autologous MSC delivery in animal Achilles tendon repair model compared to cell-free collagen control is reported. It is also demonstrate that significant improvement in histological repair of a collagenase-induced injury in the superficial digital flexor tendonitis in horses treated with autologous regenerative cells harvested from fat.

2. **Osteoarthritis**- In a caprine model of traumatic joint injury, BM-MSCs delivered intra-articularly engrafted and repair meniscal tissue, leading to a significant reduction in the progression of osteoarthritis. Multipotent MSC have been suggested as a suitable cell source for cell-based treatments for osteoarthritis due to their ability to differentiate towards chondrogenic and osteogenic lineages.

3. **Bone Repair**- The mechanisms of bone formation entail an orchestration of cellular, humoral and mechanical factors resulting in formation of skeletal bony tissues capable of controlled growth, structural response to stress, and repair of injury, uniquely without scar. The MSC is the basic cellular unit of bone formation. Secondary bone healing mimics bone formation with proliferation of MSC then their differentiation into components of fracture callus. Bone regeneration, mimics bone healing can be achieved with MSC combined with strategies of osteogenesis, osteoinduction, osteoconduction, and osteopromotion. MSC based strategies first

> employed with isolated and culture expanded stem cells in an osteoconductive carrier to successfully regenerate new bone in an critical bone defect in animal models. This bone regeneration is as effective as autologous cancellous bone. Because MSC appear to be immunologically privileged, a study using mismatched allogenic stem cell demonstrate that these cells would regenerate bone without inciting an immunologic response, documenting the possibility of banked allogenic MSC for bone regeneration (Kraus and Kirker-Head, 2006).

Continued advances in medical understanding herald the prospect of increased longevity for mankind. However, with this increased longevity and massive population of both human and animal and tremendous expand of automobiles in a congested road/ city leads to susceptibility of different diseases of skeletal system. Bone remains the second most transplanted tissues after blood. A modern treatment regime for the reconstruction and enhancement of function of fractured bone depends on autogenous or allogenic tissue grafts (Hutmacher and Sugunan, 2010). But they have their own merits and demerits. Though autogenous bone graft is the gold standard for fracture repair, but associated with donor site morbidity inflicted on the animal, the potential of infection at the bone harvested site, painful surgical procedure and the risk of injuring surrounding structures limits the use autografts for routine uses.

Novel approaches to skeletal reconstruction will result in orthopedic and reconstructive surgery undergoing a paradigram transformation by adding bone engineering to their standard treatment concepts. The most recent concept underlying tissue engineering is to combine a scaffold-matrix-, living cells and / or biologically active molecules/factors together to form a "tissue engineered construct (TEC)" to promote the repair and regeneration of bony tissue. Bone tissue engineering aims to bone defects/fractures with autologous cells and tissue without the donor site morbidity and expense associated with harvesting autogenous bone. Scaffold to support cell-based tissue engineering are critical determinants of clinical efforts to regenerate and repair the body. Bone tissue engineering requires materials that are biocompatible, well vascularized, mechanically suited for bone function, integrated with the host skeleton and support osteoinduction of the implanted cells that form new bone (Hutmacher and Sugunan, 2010). The goal of tissue engineering is to generate biologic substitutes for repair or replacement of injured tissue.

Bruder *et al.* (1998) examined the effect of cultured autologous MSC on the healing of critical sized segmental defects in the femora of adult female dogs. Autologous cultured bone marrow derived MSC that had been loaded onto porous ceramic cylinders elicited the healing of critical sized segmental bone defects in dogs.

Harris and Cooper (2004) studied to compare the osteogenic potential of bone marrow-derived, culture expanded human mesenchymal stem cells (hMSCs) adherent to different scaffolds composed of various calcium phosphates. Bone formation within synthetic HA/TCP scaffolds is measured to be 8.8% and 13.8% of the total tissue present for the 60.40% and 20.80% materials, respectively.

The excellent biocompatibility and outstanding biological properties of bioactive as well as inert ceramics have encouraged their use in bone reconstructive surgery (Maiti and Singh, 2003). Progressive improvement in the manufacturing process has allowed the production of reliable ceramic materials. Maiti and Singh (1996, 1998) also reported that presence of bone matrix, osteoinducers like bone morphogenic protein (BMP) and Transforming Growth Factor (TGF ß) is essential for utilization of different ceramics/bio- scaffold in bone reconstructive surgery.

De-Kok *et al*, (2003) designed a study to evaluate mesenchymal stem cell (MSC) based alveolar bone regeneration in a canine alveolar saddle defect model. MSCs are loaded onto hydroxyapatite/ tricalcium phosphate (HA/TCP) matrices. Scanning electron microscopic evaluation demonstrate greater than 75% MSC coverage of the HA/TCP porous surface prior to placement regardless of MSC donor. There is no histological evidence of an immunological response to autologous MSCs. Surprisingly, allogenic MSC implantation also fail to provoke an immune response. Analysis of circulating antibody levels against MSCs support the hypothesis that neither autologous nor allogenic MSCs induce a systematic response by the host. It is concluded that autologous and allogenic MSCs have the capacity to regenerate bone within craniofacial defects.

De-Kok *et al* (2005) have evaluated culture-expanded bone-marrow-derived mesenchymal stem cells (MSCs) for alveolar bone repair in terms of canine safety and potential efficacy. Neither implanted MSC –related inflammation nor ectopic osteogenesis is observed. At 21 days, bone formation is evident in all sites. After 49 days, measured bone formation is 34%, 25% and 35% for cell-loaded, cell-free and untreated sockets.

Bruder *et al* (1998) have performed preclinical studies showing the feasibility and efficacy of MSC based implants to heal large osseous defects. After confirming that syngeneic rat MSCs could heal a critical size segmental defect in the femur, it is established that human MSCs regenerate new bone of considerable mechanical integrity when implanted in an osseous defect in an immuno-compromised animal. Furthermore, bone repair studies in dogs verify that the technology is transferable to large animals and that the application of this technology to patients at geographically remote sites is feasible. These studies suggest that by combining MSCs with an appropriate delivery vehicle, it may be possible to offer patients new therapeutic options.

Reparative osteogenesis is studied by Fatkhudinov *et al* (2005) after xeno-transplantation of suspension cell graft from human mesenchymal stem cells to repair rat bone defect. On day 90, after treatment the bone regenerate is completely developed in the area of defect in animals of various groups. The newly formed bone tissue is well integrated into the bone organ.

Kraus and Kirker-Head (2006) have reviewed MSC as the basic cellular unit of bone formation. Secondary bone healing mimics bone formation with proliferation of MSC then their differentiation into components of fracture callus. Because MSC appeared to be immunologically privileged, a study using mismatched allogenic stem cells demonstrate that these cells would regenerate bone without inciting an immunologic response, documenting the possibility of banked allogenic MSC for bone regeneration.

To characterize equine bone marrow-derived mesenchymal stem cell growth characteristics as well as their adipogenic and osteogenic differentiation potential, Vidal *et al* (2006) have performed *in vitro* study. They conclude that the frequency, *in vitro* growth rate, and osteogenic differentiation potential of foals and young adult horses are similar to those documented for BM-MSCs of other mammalian species. The results have direct relevance to the use of bone marrow as a potential source of adult stem cells for tissue engineering application in veterinary medicine.

Maiti and associates (2008) have reported some preliminary findings on mesenchymal stem cell construct for osteogenesis in swine model. Mesenchymal stem cell construct are prepared after resorbable bio-ceramics fabricated with cultured bone marrow mesenchymal stem cells. Fifty per cent frontal bone defects are filled with MSC construct randomly, whereas, 50% defects are remained blank (control). Radiographic, radiomorphometric, histological and histomorphometric analysis confirmed significant osteogenesis in bone defects filled with stem cell construct than the control/blank bone defect.

Maiti *et al* (2016) used mesenchymal stem cells-seeded bio-ceramic construct for bone regeneration in large critical-size bone defect in rabbit model. The objective of the study is to determine whether the addition of recombinant human bone morphogenetic protein (rhBMP-2) and insulin-like growth factor (IGF-1) to a silica-coated calcium hydroxyapatite (HASi) - rabbit bone marrow derived mesenchymal stem cell (rBMSC) construct promoted bone healing in a large segmental bone defect beyond standard critical -size radial defects (15mm) in rabbits. An extensively large 30mm long radial ostectomy is performed unilaterally in thirty rabbits divided equally in five groups. Defects are filled with a HASi scaffold only; HASi scaffold seeded with rBMSC; HASi scaffold seeded with rBMSC along with rhBMP-2 and IGF-1 in another two groups. An empty defect serves as the control group. Radiographically, bone healing is evaluated at 7, 15, 30, 45, 60 and 90 days post implantation. Histological qualitative analysis with microCT (µ-CT), haematoxylin and eosin and Masson's trichrome staining are performed 90 days after implantation. All rhBMP-2-added constructs induce the formation of well-differentiated mineralized woven bone surrounding the HASi scaffolds and bridging bone-implant interfaces as early as eight weeks after surgery. Bone regeneration appears to develop earlier with the rhBMP-2 constructs than with the IGF-1 added construct. Constructs without any rhBMP-2 or IGF-1 shows osteoconductive properties limited to the bone junctions without bone ingrowths within the implantation site. In conclusion, the addition of rhBMP-2 to a HASi scaffold could promote bone generation in a large critical-size-defect.

Niemeyer *et al* (2010) have reported xeno-transplantation of human MSC for bone regeneration in a rabbit critical-size defect and concluded that no local or systemic inflammatory response resulting from xenogenic transplantation is observed.

Multiple studies demonstrate *in vivo* bone regeneration and repair in animal models. It has been demonstrate in several studies that BM-MSCs could be used to repair a critical bone defects as well as in non-union fracture models in different species of animals. AD-MSCs could heal a critical-size mouse calvaria defect in which there is increased bone formation and mineralization compared to controls. A human clinical case shows a dramatic regeneration of the calvarium in a young girl with severe traumatic damage.

4. **Cartilage repair**-As MSC can easily differentiate into chondrocytes; it is now routinely use for cartilage repair in horses and as well as in canines and other animal species. Scientists reported that allogenic culture expanded bone marrow-derived MSC have a chondrogenic potential and may be used successfully to repair cartilaginous defect without any significant reaction and superior to the perichondrium guided chondrogenesis.

5. **Cerebral infarction**- In a rodent cerebral infarct model, scientists demonstrate that infracted rats administered magnetically labeled AD-MSCs, two weeks after the creation of an infarct experience restoration of locomotor function compared to controls.

6. **Diabetes**: In 2001 research teams in Israel and at the Institute of Health (NIH) of USA found a way to direct the differentiation of cultured ES cells into beta pancreatic cells that made and secreted insulin. Other investigators are trying to repeat this accomplishment using adult stem cells including MSC. If this can be done, stem cells could be harvested

from each diabetic patient, stimulated to differentiate into beta cells, and then returned to the patient in the hope they will colonize the pancreas, thus curing the disease. Recently some research workers in India experimentally use MSCs for generation of beta-pancreatic islets with the aim for diabetes treatment. However, it is still in experimental stage.

7. **Neurological disorders-** There are several neurological disorders that may eventually be treatable with stem cells, including Parkinson's disease and spinal cord trauma. Dr Ronald McKay of USA has shown that mouse stem cells can repair some neural damage when injected into rates, but whether stem cells will be able to re-establish normal circuity and at the same time, remylenate the axons is yet to be determined. Dr James Thomson of University of Wisconsin is, however, confident that this will be accomplished in the near future.

8. **Cardiovascular disease-**MSCs are attractive candidate for cardiovascular repair due to their above mentioned biological properties. MSC has been shown to engraft after systemic or local administration and improve the repair of infracted myocardium. In a rat model of dilated cardiomyopathy, MSC transplantation significantly increase capillary density and decrease the collagen volume fraction in the myocardium, resulting in decrease left ventricular end-diastolic pressure. A potentially deadly form of cardiovascular disease affecting the coronary arteries is currently being treated with adult stem cells in animal models. Stem cell therapy to treat cardiovascular disease is still in a preclinical stage of development.

9. **Liver regeneration** – Bone marrow derived mesenchymal stem cells (MSCs) have the potential to inhibit the death of hepatocytes. It is found to stimulate liver regeneration via a paracrine mechanism, or it directly differentiates into hepatocytes and repopulates the injured liver. MSCs can differentiate into hepatocytes-like cells both *in vitro* and *in vivo* and can secrete trophic factors, including growth factors, cytokines and chemokines, which promote the regeneration of the impaired liver. We have evaluated mesenchymal stem cells for regeneration of liver tissue after partial hepatectomy in rats and concluded that rat bone marrow derived stem cells in combination with epidermal growth factor and conditioned media accelerated regeneration in liver after partial hepatectomy in rats (Divya, 2018).

10. **Leukomeia-** Stem cell therapy has the potential to treat all forms of leukemia with autologous transplants, thus removing the need to find bone marrow donors. Stem cells, isolated from the bone marrow of the affected

patient, can be induced to differentiate into normal white blood cells and then grown in culture to increase their numbers. Once these cells are collected, the patient's cancerous bone marrow is destroyed and the stem cell –derived blood cells are returned to the patient in order to reconstitute a healthy, cancer –free bone marrow.

11. **Skin wound repair**- It is reported that mesenchymal stem cells have tremendous role in skin wound healing. Bone marrow derived mesenchymal stem cells could promote wound healing *in vivo*, and fibroblasts originated from bone marrow are found in the repaired tissue. Allogenic mesenchymal stem cell seeded with Chitosan shows better healing potentiality than Chitosan alone in the repair of full thickness skin wound in rat model (Sandeep *et al*., 2014). Acellular fish swim bladder matrix seeded with bone marrow derived mesenchymal stem cells is found to be novel bioengineered biomaterials in full thickness skin repair (Remiya *et al*., 2014). Excellent full thickness skin burn wound healing is observed using gene embedded porcine acellular matrix with transfected mesenchymal stem cells in rat model (Tamil Mahan *et al*., 2016).

12. **Corneal wound repair**- Corneal ulceration is one of the most common ophthalmic disorders in veterinary medicine. Rabbit bone marrow derived mesenchymal stem cells seeded decellularized porcine small intestinal submucosa and porcine corneas have been evaluated for their healing potential in lamellar keratectomy wound in rabbit model. It is observed that decellularized porcine cornea seeded with mesenchymal stem cells is found to have better healing potential for the repair of corneal defect and MSCs prove as immune privileged (Sangeetha *et al*., 2014)

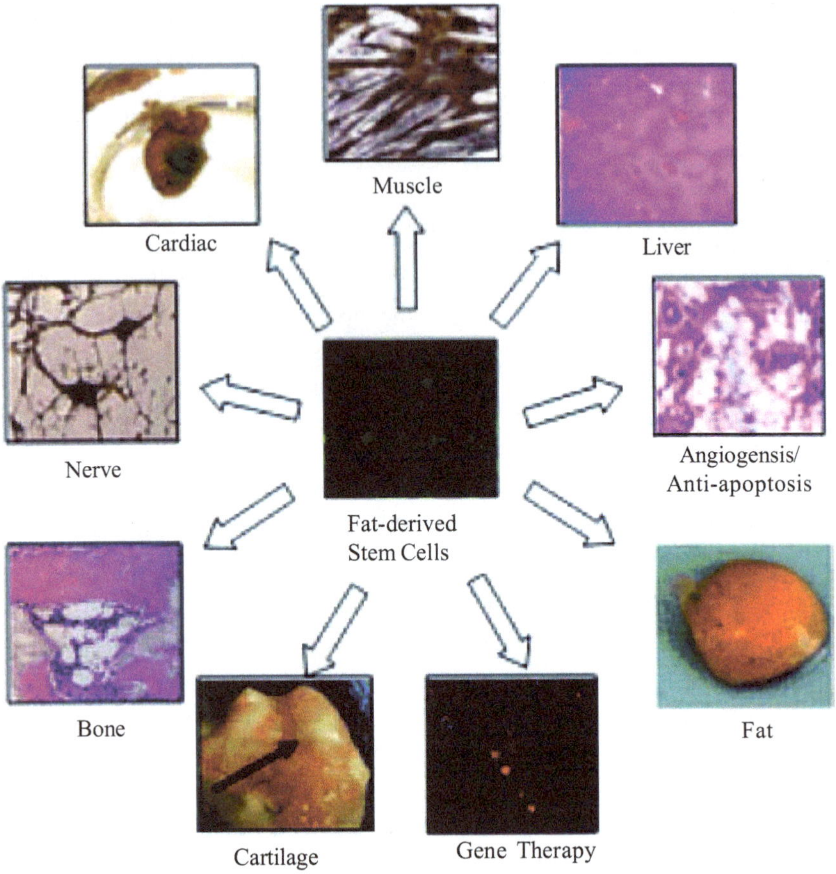

Courtesy: www.vetstem.com (Reproduced with permission)

2

Isolation, Proliferation and Morphological Characteristics of Bone-marrow Derived Mesenchymal Stem Cells (BM-MSC) from Different Animal Species

Mesenchymal stem cells are multipotential cells capable of proliferation and differentiation into osteogenic, chondrogenic and adipogenic lineages both *in vitro* and in *vivo*. Minimal criteria for defining MSC according to International Society of Cell Therapy (ISCT) are (a) they must be plastic-adherent when maintained in a standard culture conditions, (b) MSC must express some surface antigen such as CD105, CD73, CD90, CD44 and must not express CD34, CD45, CD 14, CD19, and HLA-DR, and (c) MSC must differentiate *in vitro* into osteoblast, adipocytes and chondrocytes under specific differentiating condition.

Although traditionally MSC isolated from bone marrow, more recent reports have detailed the isolation of cells with MSC characteristics from a variety of tissues including umbilical cord blood, chorionic villi of the placenta, Wharton's jelly, peripheral blood, fetal liver and lung, adipose tissue, skeletal muscle, periosteum, deciduous teeth, amniotic fluid, dental pulp, testis, synovium and the circulatory system. Bone marrow and periosteum sources are richest in young animals with their numbers diminishing, but still present in old age. It is estimated that MSCs represent approximately only 0.01 to 0.001% of the total nucleated cells within isolated bone marrow aspirate. The yield of MSCs from bone marrow varies from species to species. e.g., Canine =1 in 2.5×10^4; Feline =1 in 3.8×10^5; Murine =1 in 10.8×10^3 to 1 in 3.45×10^4 and Horses =1 in 4.2×10^3. Despite this low number, they are remains a great interest, as they can be easily isolated from a small aspirate and culture-expanded through as many as 40 population doublings to significant numbers in about 8 to 10 weeks.

One of the attractive advantage of BM-MSCs as a source of cell transplantation is their low immunogenicity. Recently, several studies have reported that BM-MSCs may be immune-privileged cells that do not elicit immune response due to an absence of their immunologically relevant cell surface markers. BM-MSCs also are known to inhibit proliferation of T lymphocytes, B lymphocytes, dendritic cells and natural killer cells.

In this chapter isolation, proliferation and morphological characterization of mesenchymal stem cells (MSC) collected from bone marrow of sheep, goat, dog, pig and rabbit is described.

Collection of bone marrow aspiration

1. From **Rabbit**: The animals are anaesthetized by intramuscular injection of Xylazine @ 5 mg/kg followed, 10 minutes later by, Ketamine @ 50 mg/kg in the thigh muscles. The area of iliac crest on either side is prepared in aseptic manner. The bone marrow aspirate is collected with the help of an 18 G bone marrow biopsy/aspiration needle from the posterior aspect of iliac crest. For the collection of bone marrow (BM), the biopsy needle is inserted through the skin and the muscle with little force. Once the needle is making contact with the bone, it is advanced by rotating it slowly until the bone cortex is penetrated. The stylet of the biopsy needle is removed and 2.5 ml of bone marrow is aspirated into a hypodermic syringe containing anti-coagulant. The biopsy needle is then removed and the same procedure is followed in the contra-lateral bone to collect another 2.5 ml of bone marrow aspirate in the same syringe. Thus a total quantity of 5ml of bone marrow aspirate is collected from each animal.

2. From **Dog**: Animals are anaesthetized with Xylazine and Ketamine at the rate of 1mg/ kg and 5mg/kg body weight IM respectively. Then the dogs are placed on lateral recumbence, so that the procedure would be easy. The skin over the site of collection is shaved and aseptically prepared. A 14-16 G bone marrow aspiration needle with an interlocking stylet is used for collection. For aspiration from the iliac crest, the greater prominence of the wing of the ileum is palpated. The needle is inserted with slow rotating movement in an angel of 45° parallel to the long axis of the ilium. Reaching the bone marrow may cause a brief reduction in pain reaction that confirms the location of the needle. After removal of the stylet, a 10ml syringe containing anti-coagulant is attached and bone marrow is aspirated.

3. From **Sheep & Goat**: Animals are sedated with Xylazine at the rate of 0.05mg/kg body weight IM. Then, the skin over the site of collection is

shaved and aseptically prepared and then the animals are placed in sitting position. A 14-16 G bone marrow aspiration needle with an interlocking stylet is used for collection. For aspiration from the iliac crest, the greater prominence of the wing of the ilium is palpated. The needle is inserted with slow rotating movement in an angel of 45° parallel to the long axis of the ilium. Reaching the bone marrow may cause a brief reduction in pain reaction that confirms the location of the needle. After removal of the stylet, a 10ml syringe containing anti-coagulant is attached and bone marrow is aspirated.

4. **From Pig:** Animals are sedated with Atropine-Azaperone-Ketamine (1:2:4 ratio) combination. The skin over the sternum is shaved and aseptically prepared and then the animals are placed in lateral recumbence. A 14-16 G bone marrow aspiration needle with an interlocking stylet is used for collection. The needle is inserted with slow rotating movement directly to the body of the sternum. After reaching into the sternum, stylet is removed and a 10ml syringe containing anti-coagulant is attached and bone marrow is aspirated.

Isolation and culture of mesenchymal stem cells (MSCs)

The marrow sample is diluted with equal amount of Dulbecco's phosphate buffered saline (DPBS) and is layered on density gradient medium at 2:1 ratio. The sample is subjected to gradient centrifuge at 3000 rpm for 30 minutes and the buffy coat containing mononuclear cells are collected carefully from the interface. The buffy coat is taken in the test tube along with the media-Dulbecco's Modified Eagle's Medium (DMEM) containing antibiotic and subjected for centrifugation for 10 minutes. Then the cell pallet are taken and diluted with same media containing antibiotic is again subjected for centrifugation for 10 minutes. The cell pallets are re-suspended, counted and plated at 2×10^5 cells/cm^2 in 25cm^2 culture flasks. The cells are maintained in Dulbecco's Modified Eagle's Medium (DMEM) containing fetal bovine serum (FBS) and antibiotics (mixture of penicillin and streptomycin) in an incubator with atmosphere of 5% CO2, 21% O2, 95% humidity at 37°C. After 4-5 days of primary culture, the non adherent cells (RBCs) are removed by changing the medium. The media are changed in every 3 days thereafter still cell confluence is observed.

Expansion of BM-MSC

Once the cells (MSCs) are attained 80-90% confluence, the cells (BM-MSCs) are passage several times to increase cell population. For that, old culture media are removed and cells are washed two times with DPBS (without Ca and Mg). Trypsin/EDTA are added into the flask and are kept at CO_2 incubator for 5-10 min for detachment of cells (confirmed by microscopic examination).Then equal volume of growth media are added to the flask and mixed gently with 5 strokes. Then it is transfer into a 15ml tube and centrifuge at 2000 rpm for 4 minutes at room temperature, supernatant are removed completely but carefully. Then the cell pellet are re-suspended in culture media and subjected for washing and cell suspension is counted. Cells are examined regularly for its viability, morphological features and confluence under high power microscope. The cells are repeatedly passage and expanded in optimal cultivation conditions in define culture medium until a pure culture is produced.

Cell staining and morphology

After the attachment of cells, they are fixed with 4% Para formaldehyde for 10 min and stained with crystal violet stain for 10 min. Excess stain is washed with tap water and after drying the plates are examined under a microscope. The polygonal, star shape and spindle shape cells are seen. In general, primary colonies of MSCs of different animal species are observed on day 4-6 post seeding. The majority of cells are round, oval-shaped growth; after 7-9 days, adherent cells are increased and gradually extended to the growth of the polygon, star or spindle-shaped. At 12-15 days, adherent cells increased significantly, and a colony formation is observed, adjacent colony and blended them into pieces for more than 70% of cells are arranged in swirling. The cells are ill-defined, elongated spindle-shaped; 15-18 days later, colony of a long spindle cells which are uniformly distributed. Cellular morphology of stem cells is varied between monolayer of round, elongated spindle-shaped with shorter/longer cytoplasmic extensions and they are grown in single cell or in cluster form. Proliferation capacity of canine and porcine MSC is much higher than other species. Mesenchymal stem cells are characterized morphologically by a small cell body with a few cell processes that are long and thin. The cell body contains a large, round nucleus with a prominent nucleolus which is surrounded by finely dispersed chromatin particles, giving the nucleus a clear appearance. The remainder of the cell body contains a small amount of Golgi apparatus, rough endoplasmic reticulum, mitochondria, and polyribosome. The cells, which are long and thin, are widely dispersed and the adjacent extracellular matrix is populated by a few reticular fibrils but is devoid of the other types of collagen fibrils.

Collection of bone marrow from different species of animal

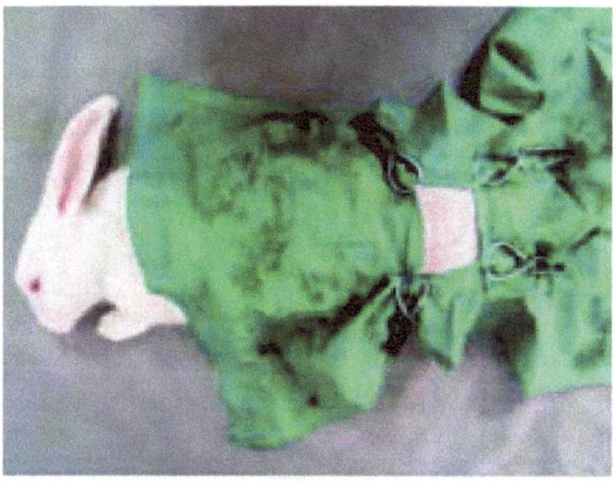

Aseptic preparation of rabbit for BM collection.

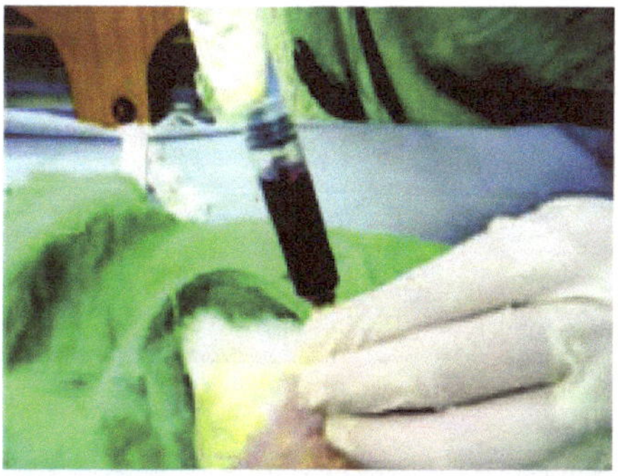

Bone marrow collection from iliac crest of rabbit.

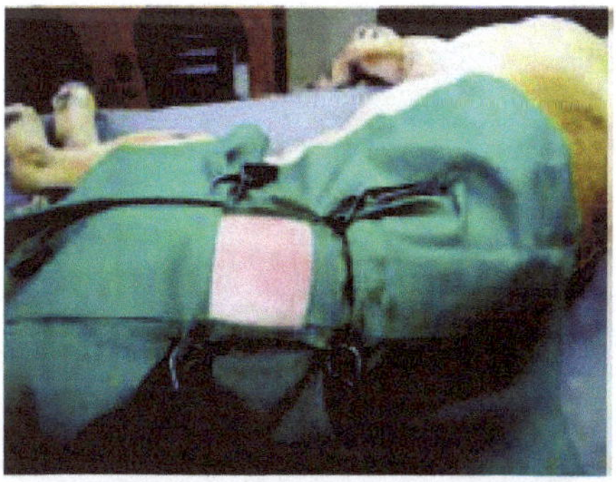

Aseptic preparation of dog for BM collection.

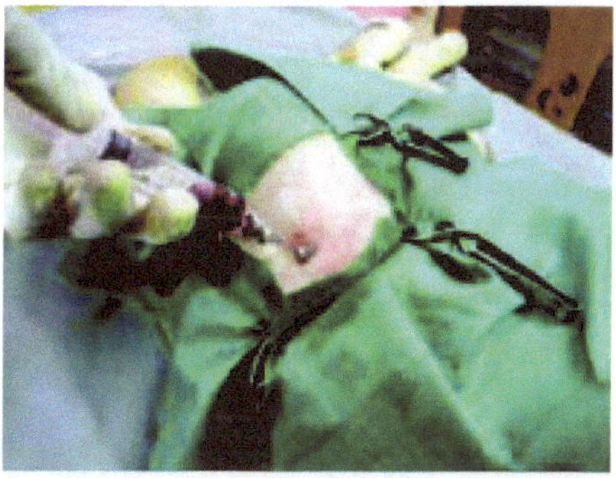

Bone marrow collection from iliac crest of dog.

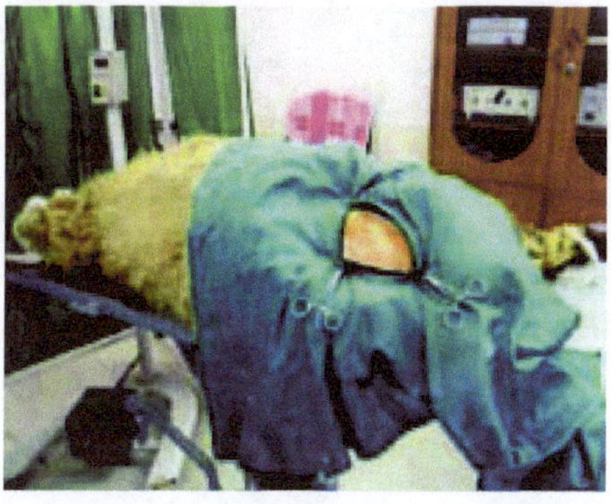

Aseptic preparation of sheep for BM collection.

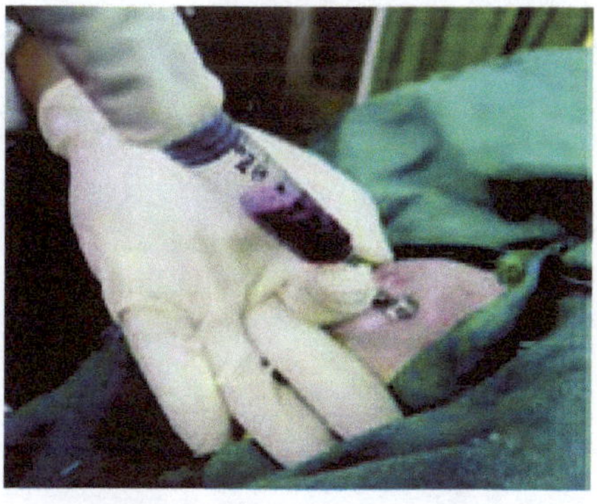

Bone marrow collection from iliac crest of sheep.

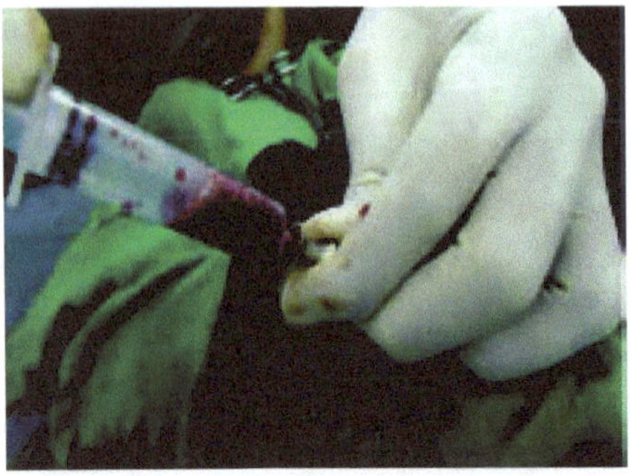

Bone marrow collection from goat

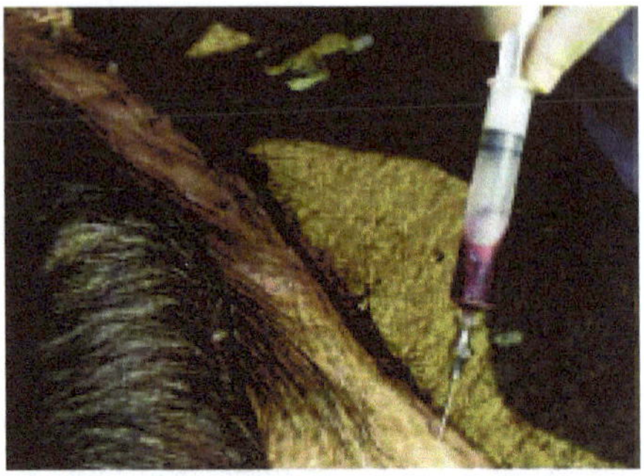

Bone marrow collection from pig

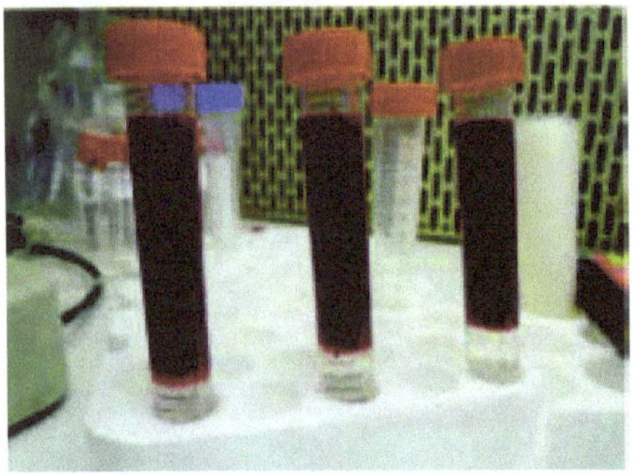

BM layered on density gradient medium

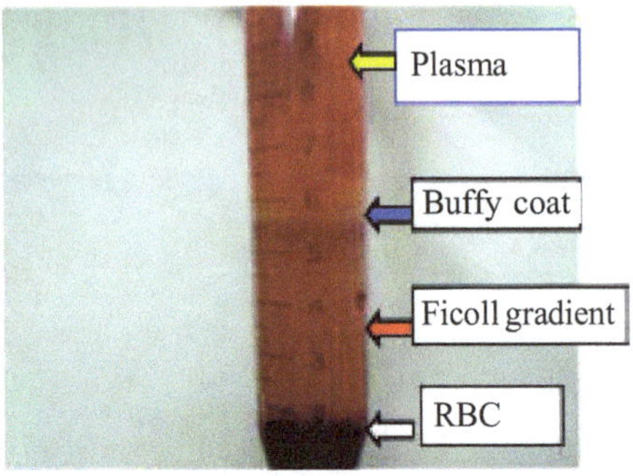

Isolation of MSC from bone marrow aspiration

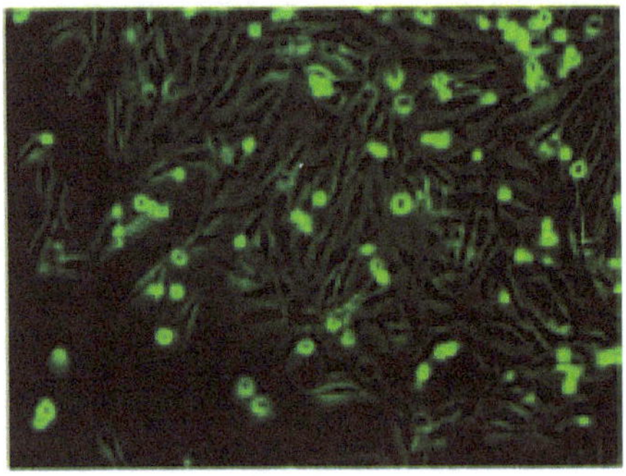

Mesenchymal stem cell of rabbit

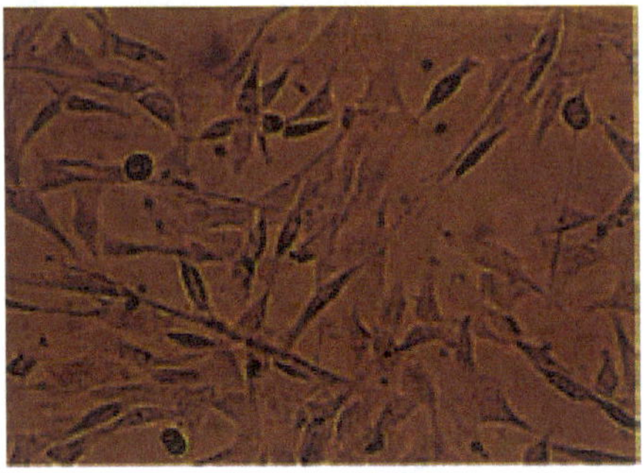

Mesenchymal stem cell of dog

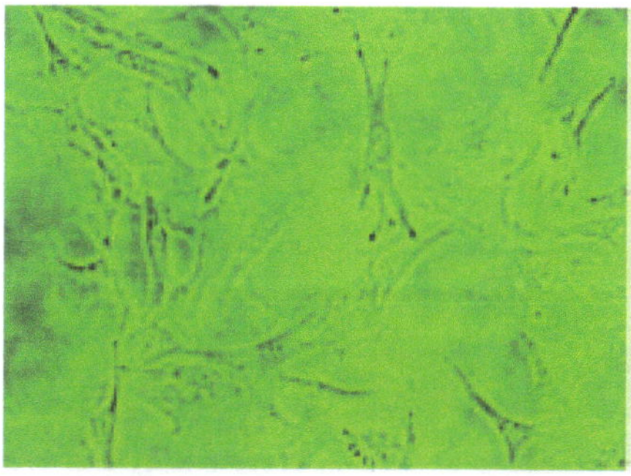

Mesenchymal stem cell of sheep

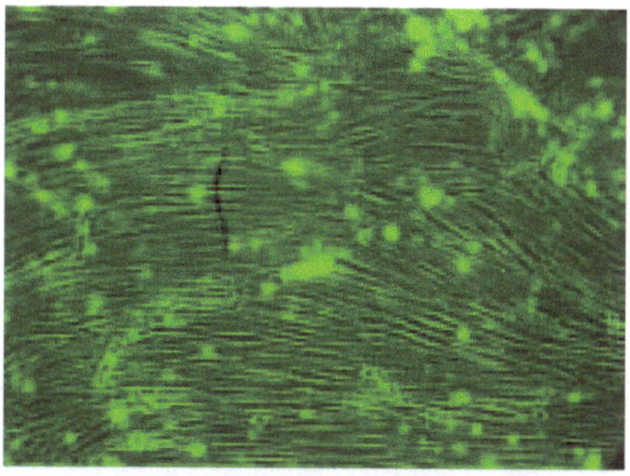

Mesenchymal stem cell of goat

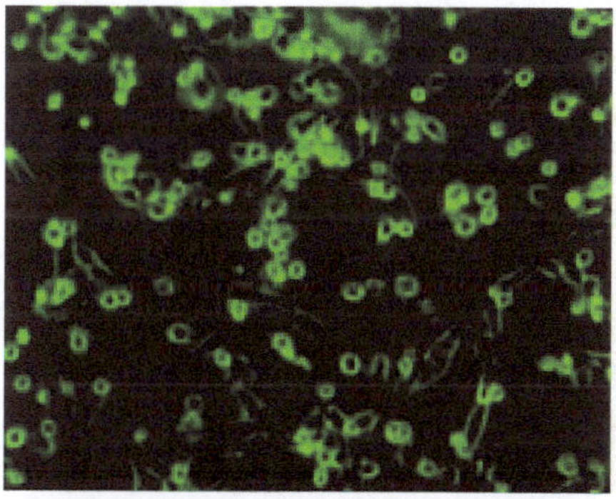

Mesenchymal stem cell of pig

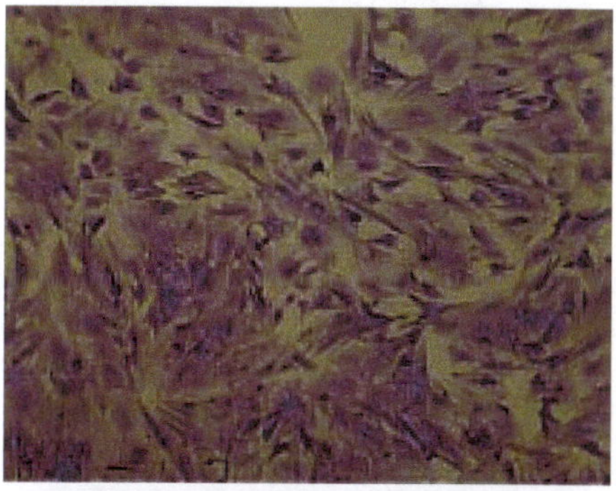

Crystal violet staining of rabbit-MSC

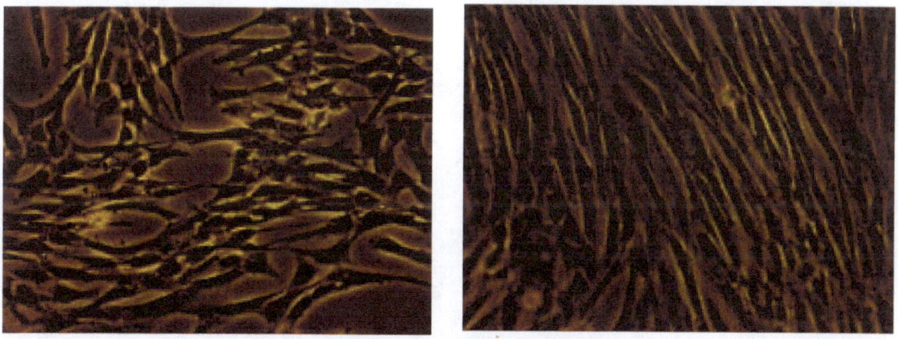

Equine Fat MSC (hrs-AT-MSC)

3

Culture, Characterization and Differentiation Potential of Rat Bone Marrow Derived Mesenchymal Stem Cells

Bone marrow contains variety of tissues including hematopoietic lineage cells and mesenchymal stem cells (MSCs). The hematopoietic cells are the major source of the blood cells in the adult body which are regulated within the microenvironment of the stromal cells of the bone marrow. MSCs are multipotent cells and can be differentiate into various cell lineage depend upon their environment and culture condition in which they are kept. Rat bone marrow derived stem cells (rBM-MSCs) have long term self renewing and capabilities of pluripotency including osteoblast, adipocytes, chondrocytes, tenocytes, muscle cells and neurogenic cells, which make them ideal source of stem cells for regeneration of injured tissue.

Bone marrow derived mesenchymal stem cells have been isolated from different species. Each species is having different culturing and growing capacity. For example human bone marrow derived stem cells are easy to harvest and maintain in culture condition whereas rat MSCs it is more difficult compared to other species. Technical difficulties in isolation limited the number of animal experiment and its required animal transplantation model for pre clinical studies. Density gradient centrifugation, plastic adherence and immunomagnetic selection like various methods are available for isolation of MSCs from bone marrow. No appropriate methods are available for selection of suitable cells. Each method has their own pros and cons. Therefore, in this chapter, combined density gradient centrifugation and plastic adherence as easy and reliable method for isolation, culture and characterization of rat bone marrow derived mesenchymal stem cell is described.

Collection of bone marrow

Ten male wistar rats aged 8-14 weeks old are prepared for collection of bone marrow. After euthanasia, animals back side are cleanly shaved and prepared aseptically. The skin incision is made on the lateral aspect of thigh and both femur and tibia from rat are taken after stripping out adherent muscles of the knee end. The collected bone is taken to laminar hood and placed in Petri dish containing DMEM (Dulbecco's Modified Eagles Medium) media with antibiotics. Both the metaphyseal region of femur is cut with scissors and hypodermic needle is inserted into the bone to aspirate the content by flushing with 1ml of complete media. The cell suspension is centrifuged at 980rpm for 5 min to concentrate the cells. The cell pellets are resuspended with 5 ml of complete DMEM medium then layered over Histopaque -1077 and centrifuged at 2500 rpm for 30 minutes. Mononuclear cells are collected from the interface by gradient centrifugation and washed with Ca+ and Mg+ free Dulbecco's Phosphate Buffer Saline (DPBS). The cell count and viability is done after addition of Trepan blue dye in the automatic cell counter then it is seeded in 1x 10^6/ml concentration in a 25 cm^2 flask. Non- adherent cells are removed after 72 hrs of cell seeding. Media is added every 3 or 4 days once until attaining confluence.

Cell Culture conditions of rat MSC

The adherent cells are supplemented with complete medium containing DMEM, 15% fetal bovine serum and 1% antibiotic mixture of 100 units/ml of penicillin and 100 μg/ml of streptomycin. The cells are maintained in a humidified chamber at 37°C which supplemented with 5% CO_2. After attaining 70-80% confluence, culture is passage with Trypsin-EDTA solution (0.25% Trypsin and 1Mm EDTA). Third passage cells are used for further differentiation studies. The culture is observed by using an inverted microscope. On initial seeding, the heterogeneous population of cells is round or oval in shape and floating over the media. MSC cells are started to attach sparsely in culture flask and other non adherent hematopoietic cells are eliminated from culture after subsequent media change. Cells are started to grow in smaller colonies after 3 or 4th day of culture. As growth continued cells are started to change their morphology from round cells to spindle shape which morphologically defined as fibroblast like cells. This fibroblast like cells are started to interconnect with other cells and monolayer confluence is attained after 15-17 days of culture. During the passaging, the morphology of cells is changed gradually and exhibit more flattened fibroblast like colonies.

Colony forming assays

For this assays, 2 cells per cm^2 are plated in 100 mm tissue culture dish and maintained up to 14 days with complete media at 37°C in 5% humidified CO_2. At the end of assay, cells are washed with DPBS and fixed in methanol for 5 minutes. Later, the cells are stained with Giemsa for 30 minutes at room temperature. Then the plates are washed with distilled water, dried and cells are counted. Colony forming assay suitable assay for assessing proliferating and colonies forming capacity of cells on third passage is measured. When cells plated at low density it is forming colonies.

Cell viability assay

The 3-(4, 5-Dimethylthiazol-2-yl)-2, 5-diphenyltetrazolium bromide (MTT) assay is used to detect the number of proliferating cells in culture based on the reduction of MTT by mitochondrial dehydrogenases. Third passage cells are plated in 96 well plate at $1x10^4$ cells / well in complete culture media for 1, 3, 7, and 14 days of incubation. Following incubation, the cells are treated with 20 µl MTT (5mg/ml) for 4 hrs at 37 °C in a 5% CO_2 incubator. After that media is removed gently without disturbing attached monolayer and dried for few minutes. 150 µl of DMSO is added to all the wells and mixed gently to dissolve the fromazan crystals without forming air bubbles. The absorbance level is measured at 570 nm wavelength in ELISA reader. The experiment is conducted in triplicate and DMSO as the blank.

Under the culture condition the proliferative capacity of rBMSC is assessed by MTT test. Cell livability / proliferation is significantly increased from day 1 to 14 (n=3) Mean ± SE 0.22 ± 0.02, 0.28 ± 0.02, 0.51 ± 0.08 and 0.61 ± 0.05 respectively

Characterization of MSC

Flow cytometric analysis of CD markers

Flow cytometric is performed in FACS caliber. The cells are centrifuged at 1200 rpm for 5 min after trypsinization then pellet is dissolved with PBS at the concentration of $1x\ 10^6$ /ml. The cells are incubated with primary polyclonal anti rat antibody against positive markers and negative markers likely CD-29, CD-90 and CD-31, CD-45 respectively at room temperature for 40 minutes. The cells are washed twice with PBS containing 2% bovine serum albumin and centrifuged at 1500 rpm for 5 min, they are resuspended with FITC labeled secondary antibody for 30 minutes at 4 °C. Cell fluorescence is evaluated in FACS caliber and data are analyzed using cell quest software.

Majority of rBMSC is expressed the surface marker positive for CD 90 and CD 29 and relatively negative for hematopoietic stem cell marker CD 31 and CD 45 which indicate that most of the cells derived from bone marrow are mesenchymal.

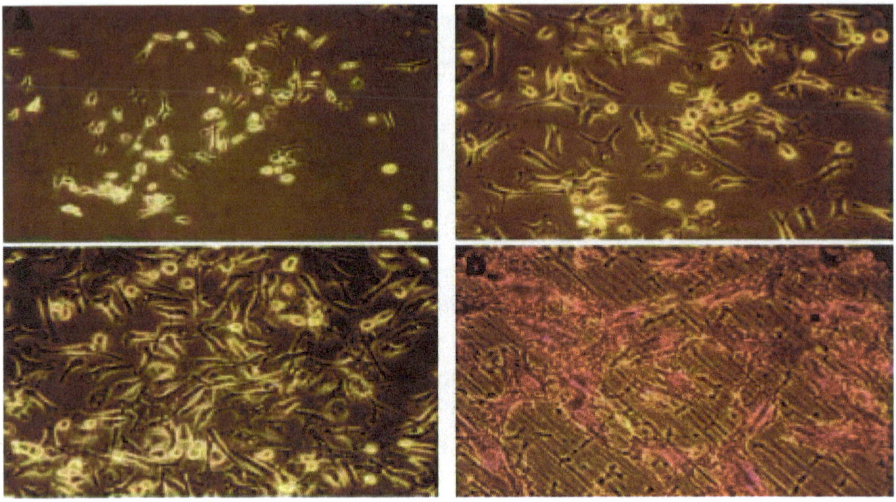

rBM-MSC growth pattern in T-25 flask. A) Cells started to change their morphology from round shape to spindle shape on day 3. B) More flattened cells on day 7. C) Getting confluence on day 15. D) Seeding on low density stained with Giemsa stain

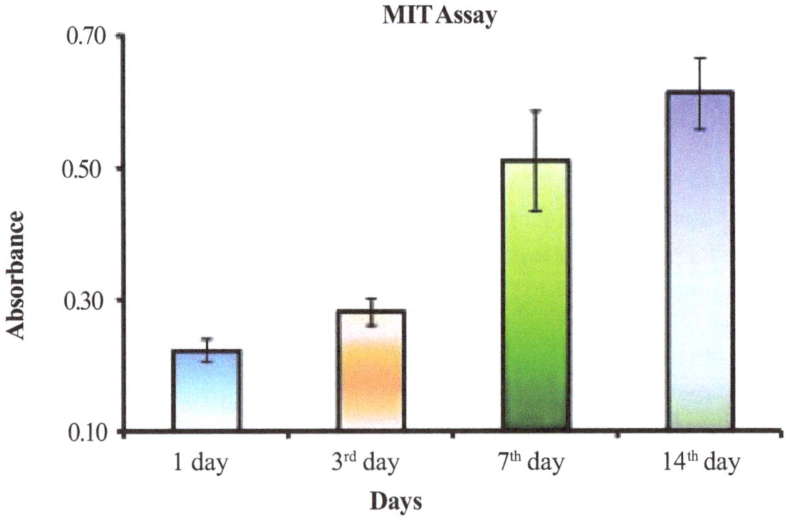

Viability /proliferation of rBM-MSC cultured in DMEM medium determined by MTT assay

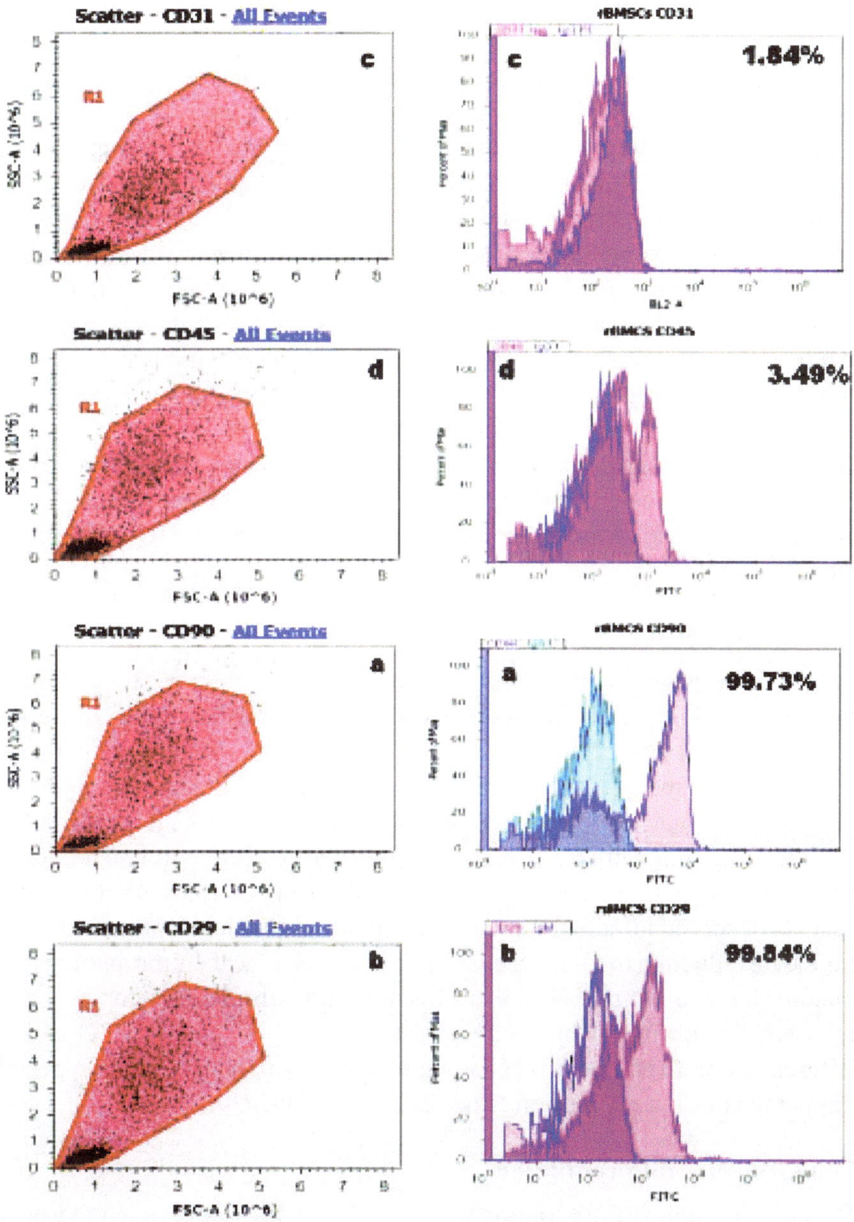

Flow cytometric analysis of negative markers (CD-31&CD-45) of rat mesenchymal stem cells (c & d). Percentage of negativity is < 5%. Flow cytometric analysis of positive markers (CD90 & CD29) of rat mesenchymal stem cells (a & b). Percentage of positivity is > 99%.

Osteogenic differentiation

Third passage cells are counted and seeded on 24 well tissue culture plate at $2x10^6$ cells per well. After attaining 80% confluence, four wells are supplemented with osteogenic differentiation medium whereas other wells are supplemented with complete medium served as negative control. Media is changed weekly twice and maintained up to 21 days. The differentiation potential of osteogenesis is evaluated by alizarin red and alkaline phosphatase staining for calcium deposition and osteogenic specific marker RunX-2 is analyzed through RT-PCR. The rMSC cells are differentiated into osteogenic lineage after 18 days of culture in osteogenic induction medium which is confirmed by presence of extracellular mineralization as evident on alizarin red staining and alkaline phosphatase staining. The positive osteogenic culture is showed more intense alizarin red staining, indicating that more calcium deposition. Control culture is showed least background staining. Alkaline phosphates staining intensity is evident in differentiated monolayer rBM-MSC compare to control cells. Further osteogenic specific gene marker Runx2 is confirmed through RT-PCR which is shown by 155 bp.

Adipogenic differentiation

To induce adipogenic differentiation, third passage cells are seeded on to 24 well plates at $2x10^6$ cells/ well. Cells are replenished with adipogenic differentiation media after reaching 80% confluence. Culture is maintained up to 3 weeks and media changed twice a week. Presence of lipid droplets in the cells indicated that positive for adipogenic differentiation which is confirmed by Oil Red O staining with 0.5% oil red O in methanol. Expression of adipogenic marker Ppar-γ is confirmed by RT-PCR. Adipocytes differentiation from rat MSC is observed after 7 days of *in vitro* culturing which supplemented with adipocyte induction medium. Cells are ability to change their morphology from spindle shape to flat one. There is a discrete lipid droplet in cytoplasm of the cells which confirmed by oil red O staining. This shows rMSC cell can differentiate in to adipocytes cells. Supplementary to above, specific gene for adipocyte (Ppar-γ) expression is detected by RT-PCR.

Chondrogenic differentiation

The chondrogenic differentiation is assessed by using stem pro- chondrogenic induction medium. Culture condition is same as mentioned in osteogenic differentiation. Culture is maintained up to 18 days. Alcian blue staining is used to assess the chondrogenic differentiation and specific marker Aggrecan is confirmed through RT PCR. Cells from third passage are subjected to chondrogenic differentiation and after attaining confluence cells are supplemented with chondrogenic induction medium. Cells are started to change their morphology (polyclonal and round) in time dependant manner compare to control which is showed on Alcian blue staining. Further this is confirmed with RT-PCR for Aggrecan specific marker for chondrocytes.

Reverse transcription polymerase chain reaction (RT PCR)

RT-PCR analysis is done to detect specific differentiation potential of rat MSC cells on standard protocol. Total RNA is isolated from differentiated rat bone marrow mesenchymal stem cells using RNeasy mini kit according to the manufacture protocols. Total concentration of RNA is measured by Nano drop 1000 spectrophotometer and measured in nanogram per micro litter. The first strand cD N A is synthesized from total RNA (1 μg) using Murine Leukemia Virus reverse transcriptase (Fermentas) for 30 minutes at 42 °C in the presence of oligo- dt primer. The PCR is carried out with cDNA template of following gene of interest RunX-2, Ppar-γ and Aggrecan.

Name	Sequence	Product size (bp)	Annealing Temp (°C)
RunX2	Forward 5'- GCCGGGAATGATGAGAACTA- 3' Reverse 5'- TTGGGGAGGATTTGTGAAGA- 3'	155	52
PPARγ	Forward 5'- CGTCCCCGCCTTATTATTCTGA- 3' Reverse 5'- CCTCGCCTTGGCTTTGGTC - 3	456	54
Aggrecan	Forward 5'- CAAGAATCAAGTGGAGCCGTGTT-3' Reverse 5'-TCAAAGTCCAGTGTGTAGCGTGT-3'	295	54

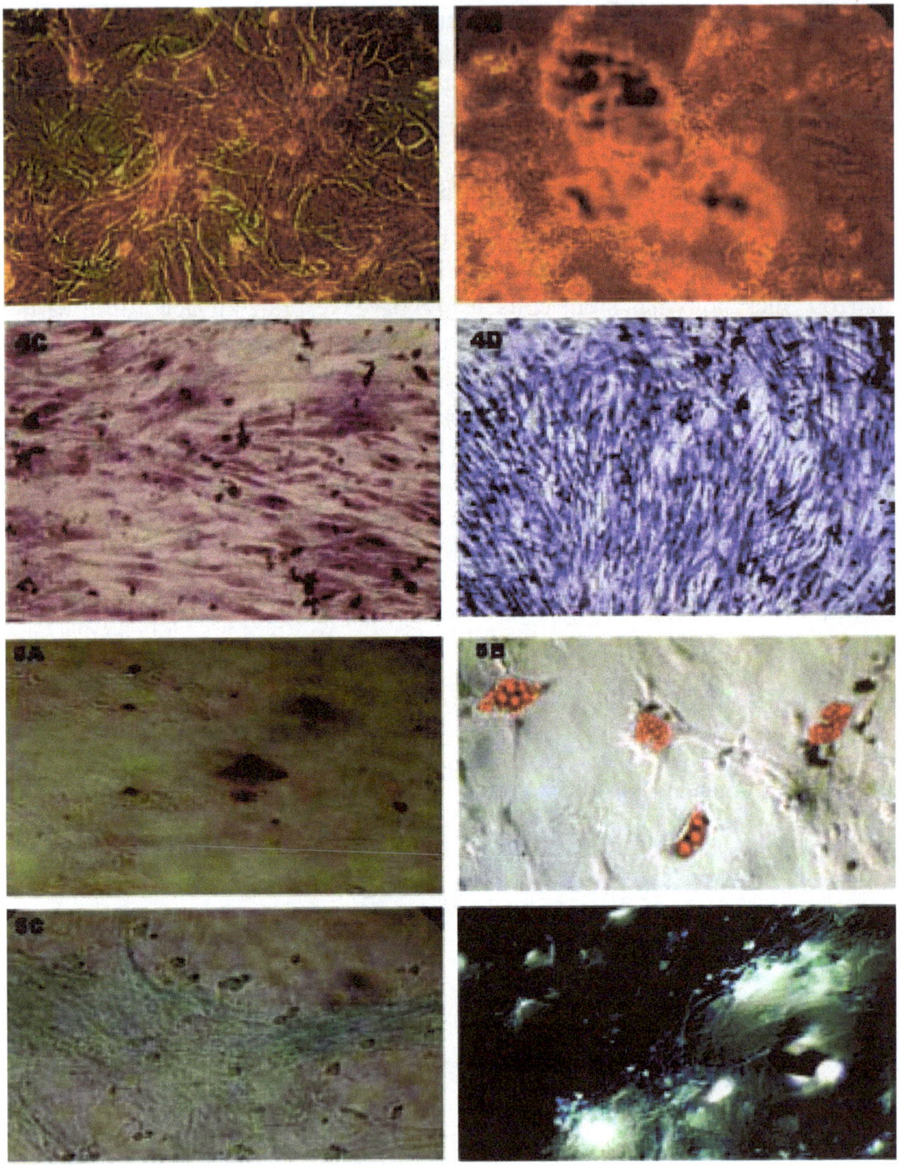

(4A) Control, (4B) Mineralization detected in alizarin red staining; (4 C) Control ALP, (4 D) rBM-MSC showed intense staining for ALP. (5A) Negative control of oil red staining, (5B) Adipocytes globules on oil red staining, (5C) Negative control Alcian blue staining, (5D) Proteoglycans production in chondrocytes positive for Alcian blue staining

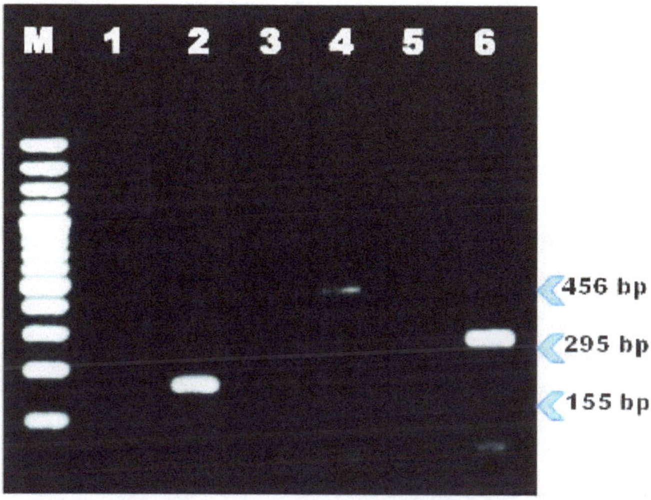

Expression of osteogenic, adipogenic and chondrogenic genes of rBMSC is measured by RT-PCR. M. Marker (100bp ladder), Lane 1: Negative control Runx 2; Lane 2: Positive for Runx 2; Lane 3: Negative control Ppar γ; Lane 4. Positive for Ppar ã; Lane 5: Negative control Aggrecan and Lane 6: Positive for Aggrecan.

In summary, the combination of density gradient centrifugation and plastic adherence is an efficient method for producing a homogenous population of rat bone marrow stromal cells. The data further demonstrated that rat MSC has ability to differentiate into highly specialized cells and each with specialized cell function. This pluripotency and self renewing capacity make them ideal source for regenerative medicine.

4

Isolation, Proliferation, Characterization of Rabbit Bone-Marrow Derived Mesenchymal Stem Cells (rBMSC)

Mesenchymal stem cells are multipotential cells capable of proliferation and differentiation into chondrogenic, osteogenic and adipogenic lineages. Minimal criteria for defining MSC according to International Society of Cell Therapy (ISCT) are (a) they must be plastic-adherent when maintained in standard culture conditions, (b) MSC must express some surface antigens such asCD105, CD73, CD90, CD44 and must not express CD34, CD45, CD 14, CD19, and HLA-DR, and (c) MSC must differentiate *in vitro* into osteoblast, adipocytes and chondrocytes under specific differentiating condition.

Although MSC is traditionally isolated from bone marrow, more recent reports have detailed the isolation of cells with *MSC* characteristics from a variety of tissues including umbilical cord blood, chorionic villi of the placenta, Wharton's jelly, peripheral blood, fetal liver and lung, adipose tissue, skeletal muscle, periosteum, deciduous teeth, amniotic fluid and synovium. Bone marrow and periosteum sources are richest in young animals with their numbers diminishing, but still present in old age. One of the attractive advantage of bone marrow derived mesenchymal stem cells (BM-MSCs) as a source of cell transplantation is their low immunogenecity. Recently, several studies have reported that BM-MSCs may be immune-privileged cells that do not elicit immune response due to an absence of their immunologically relevant cell surface markers. BM-MSCs also are known to inhibit proliferation of T lymphocytes, B lymphocytes, dendritic cells and natural killer cells.

As MSCs comprise of a mere 0.01-0.0001% of total bone marrow nucleated cells, *in vitro* cell culture expansion is inevitable to get sufficient numbers for clinical applications. Isolation technique generally is based on the adherent properties of the MSC.

In this chapter, isolation, proliferation and characterization of rabbit mesenchymal stem cells (MSC) are described.

Five skeletally mature New Zealand white rabbits of either sex between six months and one year old is used for this study.

(A) Collection of bone marrow aspiration

The animals are anaesthetized by intramuscular injection of xylazine @ 5 mg/kg followed, 5 minutes later by, ketamine @ 50 mg/kg in the thigh muscles. The area of iliac crest on either side is prepared in aseptic manner. The bone marrow aspirate is collected with the help of an 18 G bone marrow biopsy needle from the posterior aspect of iliac crest. For the collection of bone marrow (BM), the biopsy needle is inserted through the skin and the muscle with a little force. Once the needle made contact with the bone, it is advanced further by rotating it slowly until the bone cortex is penetrated. The stylet of the biopsy needle is removed and 2.5 ml of bone marrow is aspirated into a hypodermic syringe containing 0.1 ml of heparin (300U/ml). The biopsy needle is then removed and the same procedure is followed in the contra-lateral bone to collect another 2.5 ml of bone marrow aspirate in the same syringe. Thus a total quantity of 5ml of bone marrow aspirate is collected from each animal.

B) Isolation and culture of mesenchymal stem cells (rBMSC)

The marrow sample is diluted with equal amount of Dulbecco's phosphate buffered saline (DPBS) and is layered on density gradient medium -Ficoll-Hypaque in 2:1 ratio. The sample is subjected to gradient centrifuge at 3000 rpm for 30 minutes and the buffy coat containing mononuclear/nucleated cells are collected carefully from the interface in between plasma (above) and Ficoll Hypaque (below). The buffy coat containing nucleated cells is taken in the test tube added with the growth media [Dulbecco's Modified Eagle's Medium (DMEM)] containing antibiotic (Strepto-penicillin) and subjected for centrifugation for 10 minutes. Then the cell pellet are taken and diluted with same media containing antibiotic is again subjected for centrifugation for 10 minutes. The cell pellets are re-suspended, counted and plated in a $25cm^2$ culture flasks. The cells are cultured in DMEM medium containing 10% fetal bovine serum and antibiotics (penicillin G, 100U/ml; streptomycin, 0.1 mg/ml; amphotericin B, 0.25 μg/ml) in a CO_2 incubator with an atmospheric concentration of 5% CO_2, 21% O_2, 95% humidity at 37°C. The media is first changed at the third day of culture, and then every other day. Non-adherent cells are removed subsequently. The cells are achieved confluence after 10-15 days.

(C) Expansion of rBMSC

Once the cells (MSCs) are attained 80-90% confluence, they are passages several times to increase cell population. For that, old culture media is removed and cells are washed two times with DPBS (without Ca and Mg). Trypsin (0.25%) and EDTA (0.001M) is added into the culture flask and kept at CO_2 incubator for 5-10 min for detachment of cells (confirmed by microscopic examination). Then equal volume of growth media is added to the flask and mixed gently with 5 strokes. Then it is transferred into a 15 ml tube and centrifuged at 2000 rpm for 4 minutes at room temperature, supernatant is removed completely but carefully. Then the cell pellet is re-suspended in culture media and subjected for washing after which the cell suspension is counted using a hemocytometer and reseeded in flasks with pre-warmed growth medium at approximately 100,000 cells per $75cm^2$ cell culture flasks. Cells are examined regularly for its viability, morphological features and confluence under high power microscope. The cells are repeatedly passages and expanded in optimal cultivation conditions in define culture medium until a pure culture is obtained.

(D) Characterization of rBMSC

i) Flow cytometry analysis

Flow cytometry is performed in FACS Caliber equipment from the first to third passage using the anti-rabbit CD-105, CD-73, CD 44 and CD-34 and CD-45 monoclonal antibody to evaluate cell expression which are marked with goat anti mouse IgG-FITC. For determination of surface markers of BM-rMSC, first three generations of MSC are cultured, trypsinized, centrifuged and washed with DPBS two times. Then the determination of cell concentration is done and they are mixed with anti-rabbit CD-105, CD-73, CD 44 and CD-34, CD-45 monoclonal antibody. After 30 min reaction in room temperature, cells are washed with PBS two times, and mixed with FITC labeled goat anti-mouse IgG (secondary antibody), and is kept for dark reaction for 15 min and then flow cytometry is performed for expression of cell surface markers.

ii) Reverse transcription-polymerase chain reaction (RT-PCR) analysis

The expression analysis of rabbit CD105, CD44, CD45, CD34 and CD73 is done semi-quantitatively by RT-PCR using Beta Actin as reference. For that, following procedures are performed: Isolation of RNA from New Zealand white rabbit mesenchymal stem cell (r-MSC) after 3rd passage in culture cells (around 4 million) is done as per the protocol of Qiagen RNeasy plus mini kit. C-DNA preparation from isolated r-RNA is prepared by using fermentas kit. Following this PCR amplification of a 377 bp region of CD44 gene; amplification of a 533 bp region of CD73 gene; amplification of a 342 bp region of CD105 gene; amplification of a 531 bp region of CD45 gene; amplification of a 400 bp region of CD34 gene; amplification of a 432 bp region of Beta Actin gene is carried out using the following primer pairs: CD44: for 5^2-GCCTGCCCACCATGG

CTCAG-3^2 rev: 5^2-CCCGGGAGACC CACTGC TCA-3^2; CD73: for 5^2-CACTCAGTCATGCC GCTTTA-3^2 rev 5^2-CGCTGATATCTTGCTCACCA-3^2; CD105: for 5^2-CCGGCGAATACTCTCTCAAG-3^2 rev 5^2-AGGTCAGGT TCAGGATGGTG-3^2; CD45: for 5^2-TCCCGCCGACACAGCTCTCA-3^2 rev 5^2-GGCCTGGCATTCACGTCCCA-3^2; CD34: for 5^2-TAGGGCTCAG TGCCTGCTGCT-3^2 rev 5^2-GCCGTTTCTGGAGGTGGCCT-3^2; Beta Actin: for 5^2-AAGGACCTGTACGCCAACAC- 3^2 rev 5^2-CACCTTCACCGTT CCAGTTT-3^2.

The following 3 step programme is optimized by the trial of various annealing temperatures.

PCR Programme for amplification

Sl.No.	Steps	Temperature for amplification	Time
1.	Initial denaturation	95°C	5 min.
2.	Cyclic denaturation	95°C	45 sec
3.	Cyclic Annealing 55°C		45 sec
4.	Cyclic extension	72°C	45 sec
Steps 2 to 4 were repeated 35 times			
5.	Final extension	72°C	10min.
6.	Storage	4°C	for ever

After the execution of PCR programme, the PCR product is stored at 4°C. The amplicon are checked by 1% agarose gel electrophoresis at 90 V for 45 minutes. The amplified products are visualized under gel-documentation system and image is captured and saved for further analysis.

Osteogenic differentiation

Undifferentiated cells are induced towards the osteogenic lineage. Putative MSC is seeded in six well plates at a density of approximately 3000 cells/cm^2 and cultured in expansion media till it reached 90 -100% confluence. Osteogenic differentiation is hereafter induced by culturing the cells for 20 days in osteogenic induction medium (OS) consisting of 100nM dexamethasone, 10mM β-glycerophosphate, and 0.05 mM L-ascorbic acid-2-phosphate and 10% FBS in low glucose DMEM. As a negative control an equal number of wells are maintained in expansion media for 20 days. The media in both groups are completely replaced every 4 days. The cells are cultured at 37°C in a CO_2 incubator at 5% CO_2 and maximum humidified environment. The presence/ differentiation of osteoblasts is confirmed by mineralization staining (Alizarin Red S staining) and alkaline phosphatase activity.

Alizarin Red S staining

Alizarin Red S, staining of calcium deposits is done by carefully aspirating the medium from each well so that the cells are not aspirated. The cells are fixed by incubating in ice-cold 70% ethanol for 5 minutes at room temperature, before carefully aspirating the alcohol and rinsing twice (5 minutes each) with water. The pH value of the Alizarin Red S solution is adjusted to a 4.1-4.3 with ammonium hydroxide prior to the procedure. The water is aspirated and 1 ml of 2% Alizarin Red S solution is added. The plate is incubated at room temperature for 10 minutes, before removing the Alizarin Red S solution and washing the wells five times with 2 ml water. Water is added to wells to prevent the cells from drying and the plates are visualized under bright field microscopy.

Alkaline Phosphatase assay

Alkaline phosphatase (ALP) assay is performed as a routine marker for osteogenic differentiation of MSCs, and normally, intracellular ALP activity increases rapidly during *in vitro* osteogenesis. The assay for expression of the alkaline phosphatase in BM-rMSC is conducted after fixation of cells with ethanol using alkaline phosphatase staining kit. The cell layer is washed with distilled water and incubated with the staining solution prepared according to the instruction manual at room temperature for 20 min in the dark. The colorimetric reaction is stopped by washing with dist water and the cells are stored in PBS, until the analysis with bright field microscopy.-ALP can hydrolyze Naphthol AS-MX phosphate to Naphthol AS-MX, and the latter combines with fast violet B salt to form the bluish purple, insoluble, granular dye deposit, which indicates sites of ALP activity.

Adipogenic differentiation

The adipogenic differentiation potential of rBMSCs is evaluated by culturing in Mesencult basal medium with 10% of FBS containing isobutilmetilxantine, indomethacin, dexamethasone and insulin. After 8 days of induction, cells are stained with OIL Red O.

Chondrogenic differentiation

The chondrogenic differentiation of rBMSCs is achieved for 3 weeks with DMEM, dexamethasone, ascorbic acid-2-phosphate, sodium pyruvate, L-proline and transforming growth factor-β3. The control cells are cultured in the same medium in the absence of TGF-β3. The medium is changed 3 times per week. For Alcian Blue staining, cells are rinsed once with DPBS, and is fixed with 4% formaldehyde solution for 30 min. After fixation, rinsed wells with DPBS and stained cells with 1% Alcian Blue solution. Then rinsed wells 3 times with 0.1

N HCl, added distilled water to neutralize the acidity, visualized under light microscope, and captured images for analysis.

Colony forming unit-fibroblast (CFU-F) assay and colony forming unit-osteoblast (CFU-OB) assay

For CFU-F assay, 1×10^6 bone marrow nucleated cells per 60-mm dish are seeded and cultured at 37 °C in 5% CO_2 for 12 days with media change every 2 days, followed by Giemsa staining. The numbers of CFU-Fs are counted under a microscope. For CFU- OB assay, 1×10^6 bone marrow nucleated cells per 60-mm dish are seeded and cultured for 21 days in differentiation medium. Media is changed on every 2 days. Alizarin red staining is done to identify the mineralized bone matrix of osteoblast differentiated colonies. These colonies are enumerated and designated as CFU-OB colonies.

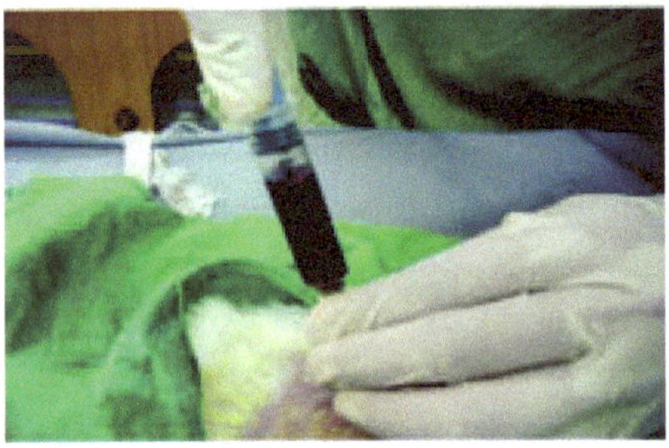

Bone marrow aspiration from iliac crest

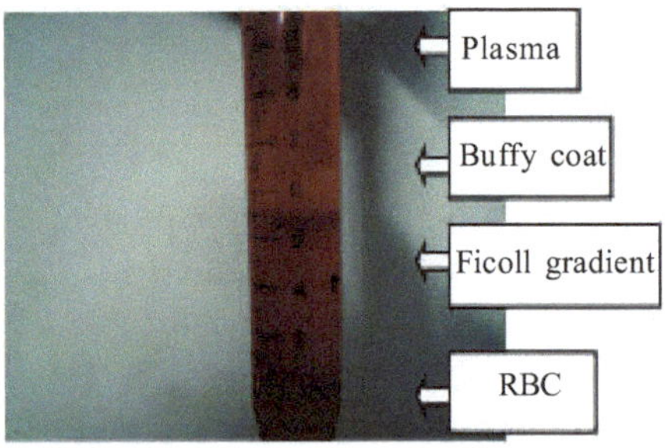

Gradient centrifugation of bone marrow

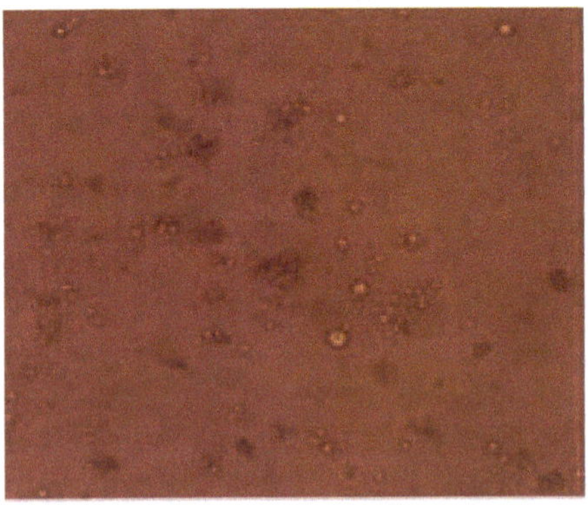

Day 0 showing floating of round cells

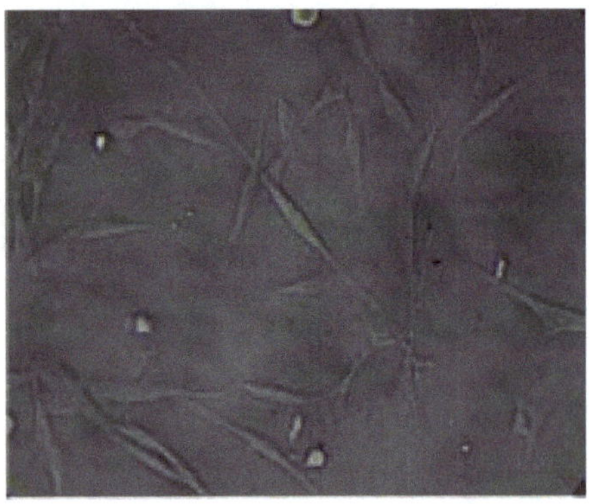

Day-5 showing spindle and polygonal cells

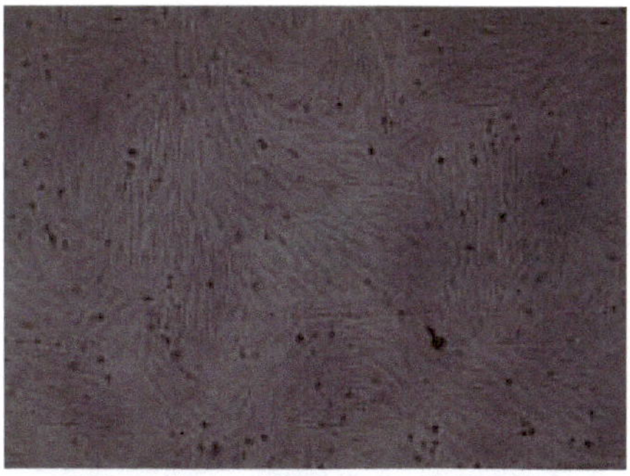

P2 cells: uniform spindle shape morphology

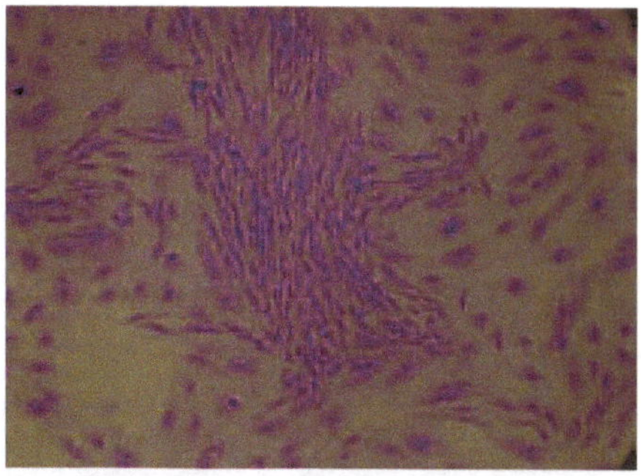

Crystal violet staining of rBMSC

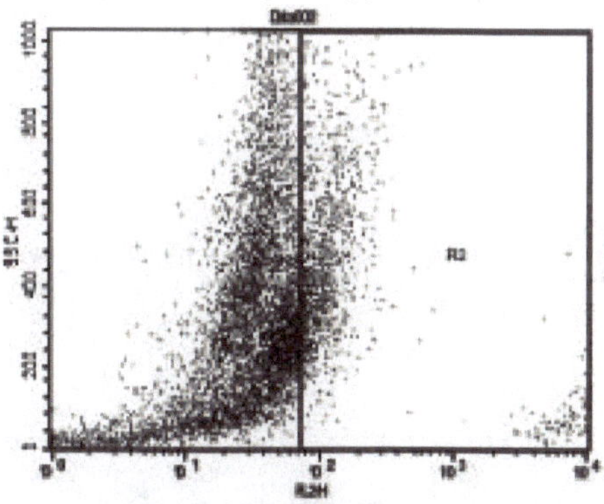

Positive expressions of CD-105

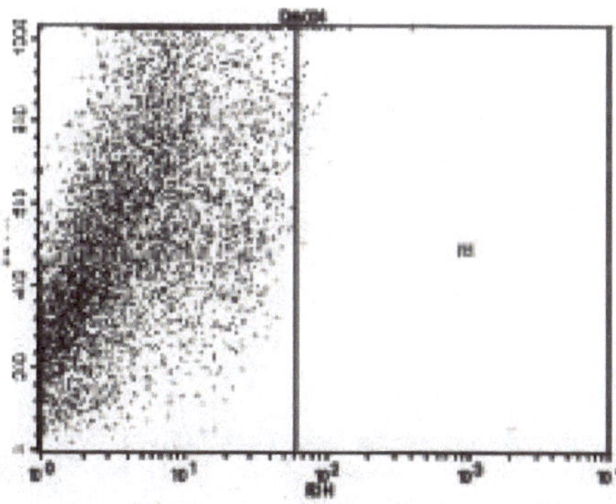

Negative expression of CD-34 in FACS

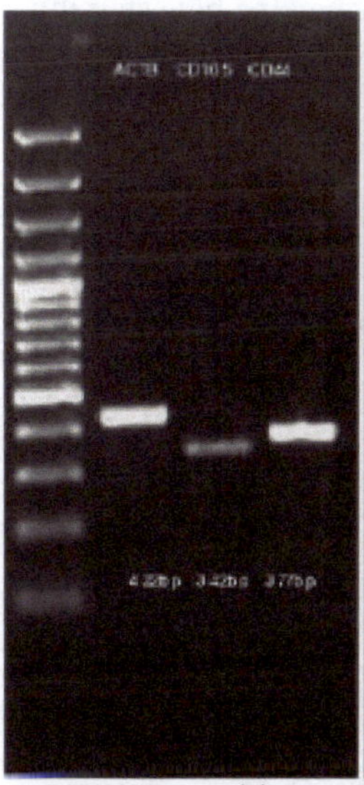

RT-PCR- positive expression for CD 105 & CD 44

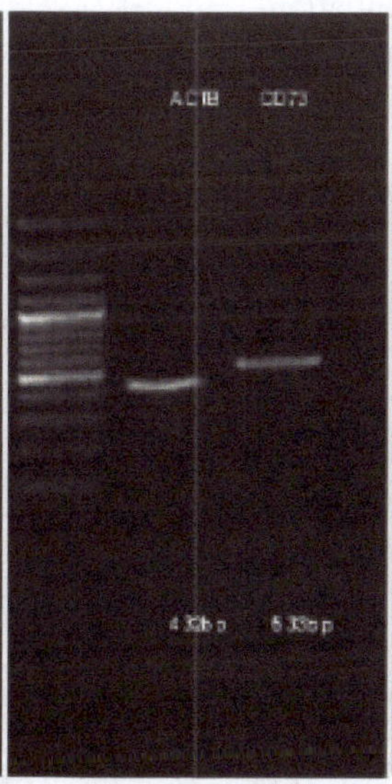

RT-PCR showing positive expression for CD 73

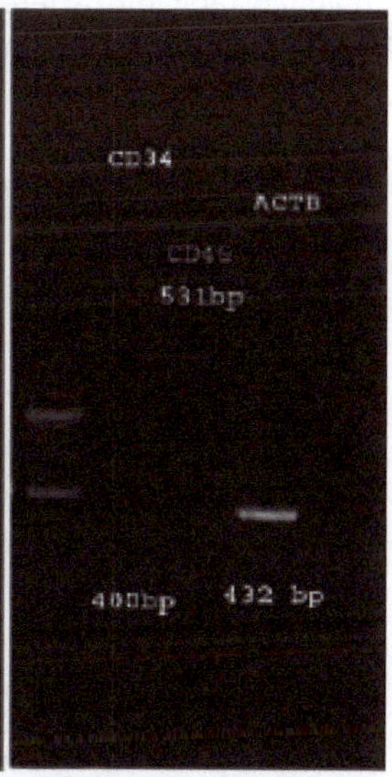

RT-PCR showing negative expression for CD 34 & CD 45

Alizarin red staining showing orange red calcium deposits

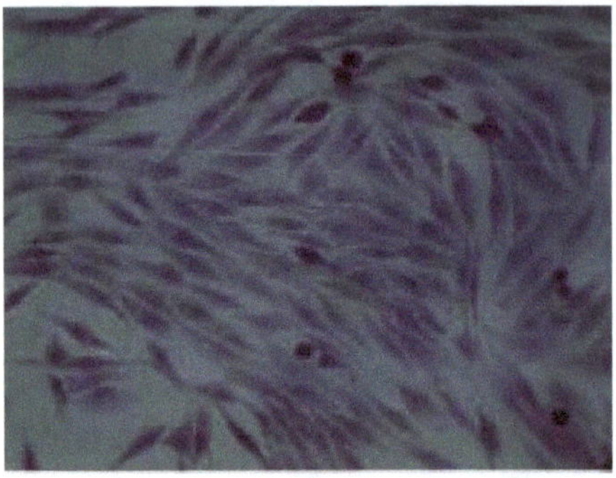

Control culture for alizarin red staining showing absence of calcium deposits

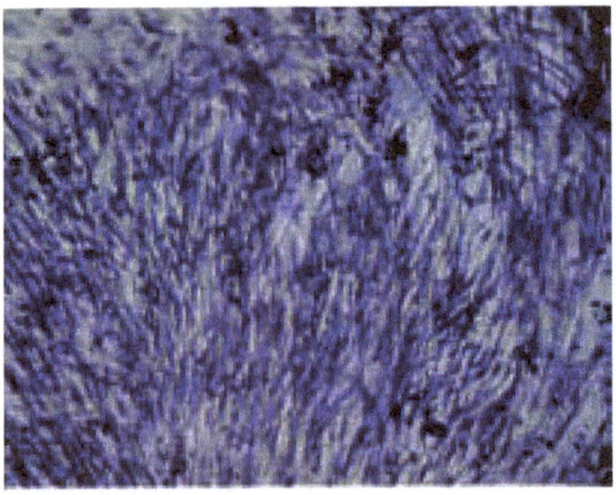

Alkaline phosphatase staining of MSCs following osteogenic differentiation showing bluish purple granular dye deposits.

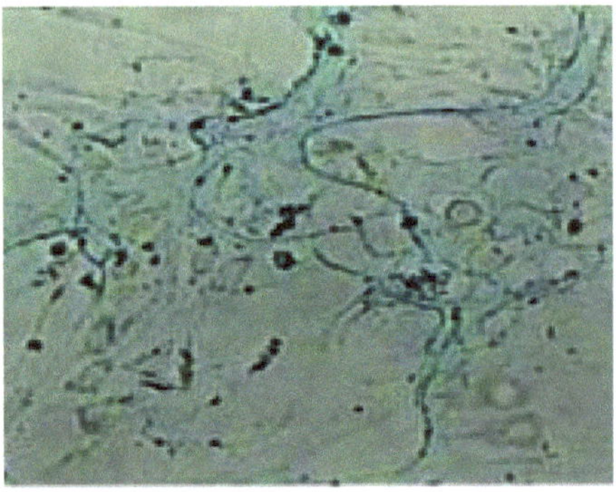

Chondrogenic differentiation of rBMSCs showing blue staining with Alcian blue stain

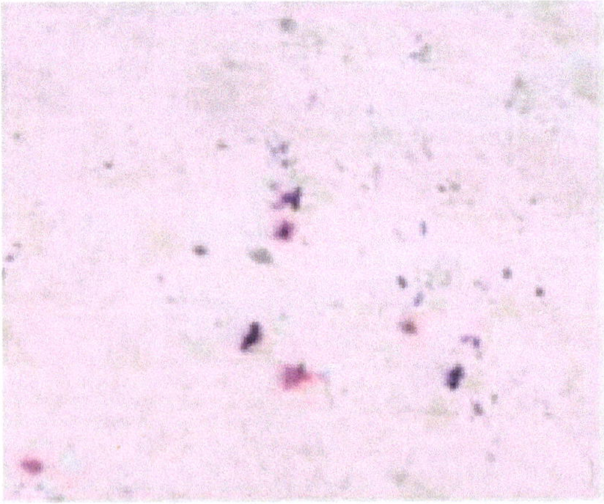

Adipogenic differentiation of rBMSCs showing deep red stained oil droplets with Oil Red O staining

5

In vitro Osteoinduction Potential of A Novel Silica Coated Hydroxyapatite Bioscaffold Seeded with Rabbit Mesenchymal Stem Cell

The knowledge and principles from interconnected disciplines of bioengineering, material science and life sciences are combined in tissue engineering with the aim of developing a construct that can wholly or partly restore/maintain/augment the function of a damaged tissue or organ. Tissue engineering construct generally comprises cells on a suitable scaffold. The ultimate functionality of a tissue engineering construct is mainly dependent on the cell behavior on scaffolds. The proliferation and cell viability on scaffolds varies from one cell type to another and from one species to another. So it is important to investigate individual cell-scaffold combinations.

The similarity in structure and composition to bone mineral, osteoconductive properties, ability to integrate with the bony tissue and absence of immune response makes hydroxyapatite [Ca_{10} $(PO_4)_6(OH)_2$] the choice of calcium phosphate biomaterial with only disadvantage of slow rate of resorption. On contrary, silica–calcium phosphate composite in comparison to calcium phosphate is rich biomaterials having a faster resorption rate. Studies have shown that coating of hydroxyapatite with a calcium silicate containing layer encourages cell proliferation and osteogenic differentiation of human bone marrow-derived stromal cells.

In this chapter a composite scaffold (calcium silicate, hydroxyapatite and tricalcium phosphate), namely HASi with elements in the following percentages: 66.36 % - calcium, 25.35 % - phosphorus and silicon - 8.29 % and porosity of 50 – 500 µm is undertaken to evaluate the rBMSC proliferation and differentiation properties *in vitro* with the aim of assessing cytocompatibility of HASi and rBMSC in terms of cell attachment, cell morphology, cell proliferation and osteogenic differentiation.

rBMSC isolation and culture

Bone marrow aspiration, isolation and culture of rBMSC are done as describe in previous chapter.

Quantification of mesenchymal progenitors (CFU-F Assay)

For CFU-F assay, 1×10^6 bone marrow nucleated cells per 60-mm dish are seeded and cultured at 37 °C in 5% CO_2 for 12 days with media change on every 2 days, followed by crystal violet staining. The numbers of CFU-Fs are counted under a microscope.

Quantification of osteoblasts (CFU-OB Assay)

For CFU- OB assay, 1×10^6 bone marrow nucleated cells per 60-mm dish are seeded and cultured for 21 days in differentiation medium (α-MEM containing 10% FBS, 1% penicillin/streptomycin, 50 μg/ml L-ascorbic acid and 2.0 mM b-glycerophosphate). Media is changed on every 2 days. Alizarin red staining is done to identify the mineralized bone matrix of osteoblast differentiated colonies, designated as CFU-OB colonies.

Osteogenic differentiation

Undifferentiated cells are induced towards the osteogenic lineage. Putative MSC is seeded in six well plates at a density of approximately 3000 cells/cm^2 and cultured in expansion media till it reached 90 -100% confluence. Osteogenic differentiation is induced by culturing the cells for 20 days in osteogenic induction medium (OS) consisting of 100nM dexamethasone, 10mM β-glycerophosphate, and 0.05 mM L-ascorbic acid-2-phosphate and 10% FBS in low glucose DMEM. As a negative control an equal number of wells are maintained in expansion media for 20 days. The media in both groups is replaced completely on every 4 days. The cells are cultured at 37^{0}C in a CO2 incubator at 5% CO2 and maximum humidified environment. The presence/differentiation of osteoblasts is confirmed by mineralization staining (Alizarin red S staining) and alkaline phosphatase (ALP) activity.

Fluorescent staining of rBMSC-scaffold constructs

For assessment of cell viability and attachment on scaffold, the cell–scaffold constructs are rinsed twice with sterile PBS and submersed in 3mL of PBS. CFDA-SE is then added to the PBS and incubated for 15 minutes at 37^0 C to label live cells green by labeling intracellular esterase as recommended by the manufacturer. They are rinsed twice again with PBS. Propidium iodide (PI) (20μg/ml, Molecular Probes) in PBS is added for 2 min at room temperature followed by washing with PBS. All steps are performed in the dark and samples are then viewed under a fluorescence microscope.

Scanning electron microscopy (SEM) study

Attachment properties and morphology of rBMSCs from third passage are assessed on HASi blocks of 0.3x0.2x0.1cm dimension. For this, the scaffold blocks are coated with fibronectin for 24 h and then surface seeding of third passage rBMSCs is done with 1x 10^6 cells per mL of DMEM medium containing 10% fetal bovine serum and antibiotics in six well plates followed by incubation at 37^0C in a humidified 5% CO_2 environment. Unseeded scaffolds are also maintained in the same culture conditions as control. The cell-loaded scaffolds and control are rinsed with PBS after 3 and 17 days of cell seeding respectively, and fixed with glutaraldehyde 2.5% for 1 h. Then the scaffolds are dehydrated with a graded ethanol series and incubated for 10 minutes in hexamethyl-disilazane (HMDS) and dried overnight in desiccators, and are gold coated. They are observed under scanning electron microscope.

Evaluation of calcium crystals

The ability of cells to produce mineralized matrix and calcium crystals is a key factor for bone regeneration. To determine the formation of calcified extracellular matrix deposition due to mineralization phenomena, a histochemical technique is used. Cells harvested from trypsinized scaffolds are fixed in 70% ethanol followed by washing with PBS and stained with 1 % alizarin red solution for 2 min. They are washed again with PBS and observed under a light microscope.

Histological evaluation

The decalcified scaffolds with Goodling Stewart's solution after day 17 post-seeding is maintained in the same culture conditions as for SEM analysis. They are subjected for histological study with H & E staining to evaluate the bone formation ability.

Result

Bone marrow collection from rabbits is carried out as per the standardized procedure. The mesenchymal stem cells are successfully isolated, cultured and propagated from all the aspirated bone marrow samples. Third passage of rBMSC is used for seeding in HASi scaffold.

From CFU-F assay, 52±2.3 (mean ± SD) colonies of fibroblast are obtained from three different trials and from CFU-OB assay, 49±2.6 (mean ± SD) colonies of osteoblasts are obtained from an initial seeding density of 1 X 10^6 cells from buffy coat and third passage respectively in 60 mm culture dish.

To characterize unique differentiating property of rBMSCs and mineral deposition, osteogenic differentiation is performed in monolayer culture for 3 weeks. The cells are changed from a fibroblastic appearance to a more cuboidal appearance at day 9 of culture. Proliferation and differentiation of control and OS cultures are compared using inverted microscope. In both cultures, cells are proliferated and reached almost complete confluence at day 9. In OS cultures, nodular aggregates of cells became evident at day 9 of culture and increased up to 21 days. These aggregates are characterized by deposits of amorphous material. In control cultures aggregates are not observed and deposits are also lacking. The OS cultures are stained positive (orange red) with alizarin red S stain for mineral (calcium) deposition in their newly formed matrix. Alizarin red positive nodular aggregates present at day 21 are larger and stained more intensively, indicating that a more extensive calcium deposition has occurred. In the control wells, adherent monolayer of swirling spindle shaped cells became over confluent without any cell aggregates and is stained negative for mineral deposition. ALP activity or expression is higher in osteogenic differentiated cells than control culture. In positive cases, the nucleus of MSCs takes bluish-purple colour.

Fluorescent staining of rBMSC-scaffold construct reveals that the live cells emitted green fluorescence. On day 3 post seeding, no dead cells are seen.

SEM observation of the seeded scaffold on day 3 post-seeding shows stem cell attachment on the surface of HASi. They have a wavy surface and the attachment is close but not tight. On day 17 post-seeding, the attached stem cell shows expansion and proliferation to form cell sheet-like structure with strong anchoring to the scaffold surface by footpads. There is matrix deposition in the form of crystals over and around the attached stem cells. The cells are seen closely attached to the side wall of the pores. The panoramic view of calcium matrix deposition by the attached cells is similar to snow covered caves. The adjacent crystals physically entangled to form a strong interconnected network that shows similarity with calcium orthophosphate. The control HASi is maintained in same culture conditions for the same time period as 17 days post-seeding samples, do not show any crystal deposits.

Trypsinization and subsequent alizarin red staining of the crystals deposits from day 17 post-seeding sample of HASi shows intense red staining indicative of presence of calcium. The histological sections stained with H& E staining shows pink stained areas indicative of beginning of early new bone formation.

Scaffolds can potentially replace damaged or diseased tissues. They may be used for enhancing the *in vivo* viability and differentiating potential of stem cells. Hydroxyapatite is the most commonly used synthetic biomaterial for bone defects because of its osteoconductive properties, ability to integrate with bony tissue and minimal immune response but with the drawback of slow resorption rate. The faster resorption rate of silica coated hydroxyapatite is due to the greater dissolution of Si ions.

Mesenchymal stem cells are known to have the ability to undergo osteogenic differentiation under suitable conditions. In this study the *in vitro* conditions for proliferation and differentiation of mesenchymal stem cells to osteoblastic lineage is established. *In vitro* fluorescent staining of the seeded scaffold proves that there is attachment of mesenchymal stem cells on the HASi scaffold on day 3 post-seeding and these cells are alive. SEM examination shows that on day 3 post-seeding, there is attachment of mesenchymal stem cells.

Conclusion and clinical relevance

Bioscaffold HASi has the potential to induce osteogenic differentiation of rBMSCs resulting in calcium matrix deposition in the absence of osteogenic induction medium. The rBMSC-HASi construct may be a promising bone substitute for autograft in non-healing and delayed fracture healing with potential bone loss. Further research is needed for understanding the cellular and molecular mechanisms of osteoinduction of the stem cell construct noticed in this study. Further research is also emphasized to investigate individual cell-scaffold combinations and investigate proliferation, viability and osteogenic differentiation of BMSC of different animal species on HASi scaffold for one ideal stem cell-based tissue engineering.

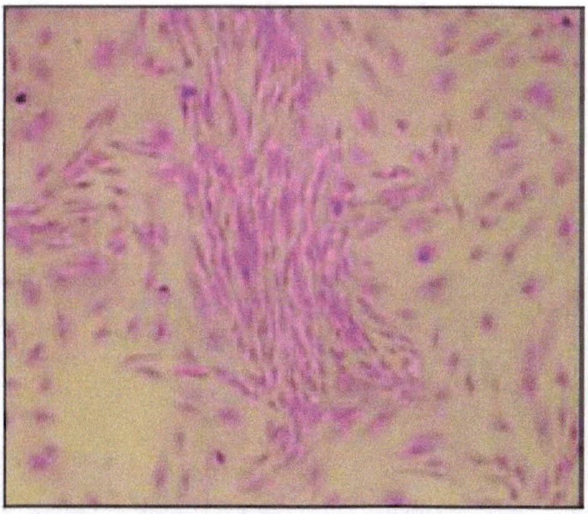

Crystal violet staining of rBMSC

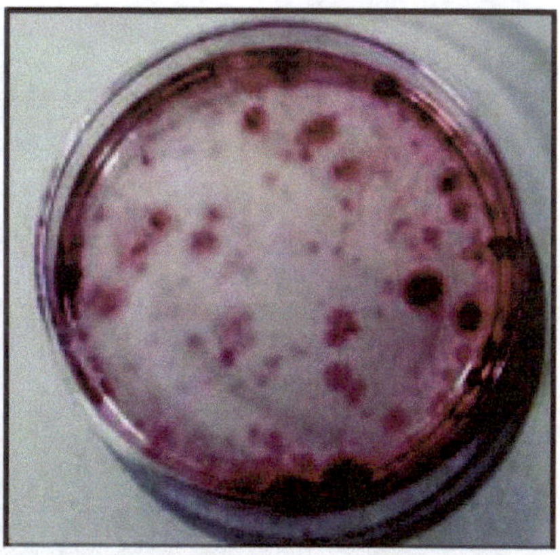

Colony forming units of osteoblasts

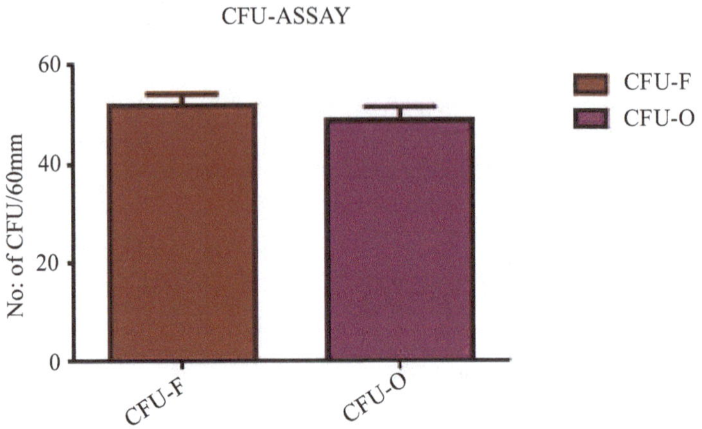

Histogram showing number of CFU of fibroblasts and osteoblasts (mean ±± SD) from an initial concentration of 1x 10^6 cells

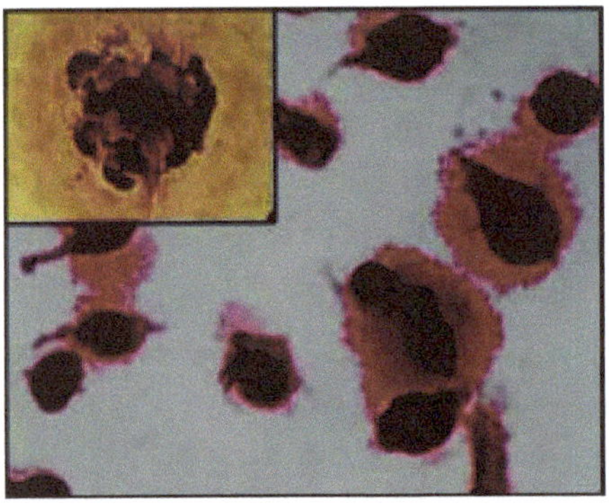

Orange red staining calcium nodules representing osteoblastic differentiation of rMSC

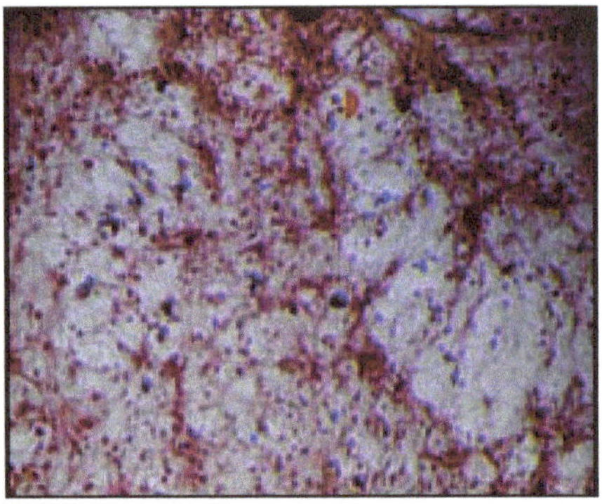

Osteoblast with bluish purple nucleus after ALP staining (200X)

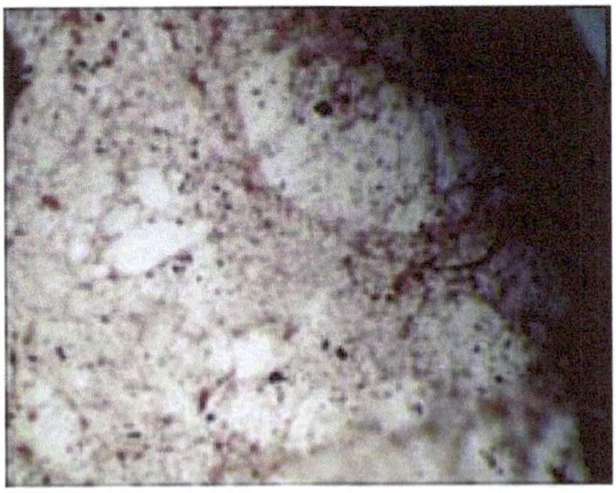

Control well after ALP staining

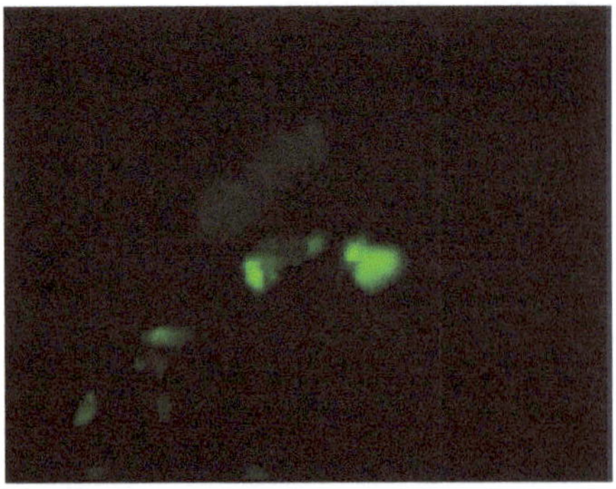

Live cells emitting green fluorescence on day 3 post-seeding on the HASi scaffold

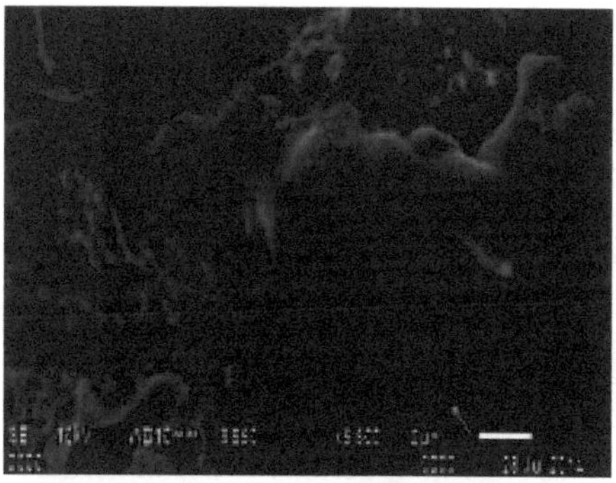

SEM analysis of rBMSC seeded HASi on day 3 showing attachment of stem cell (arrow)

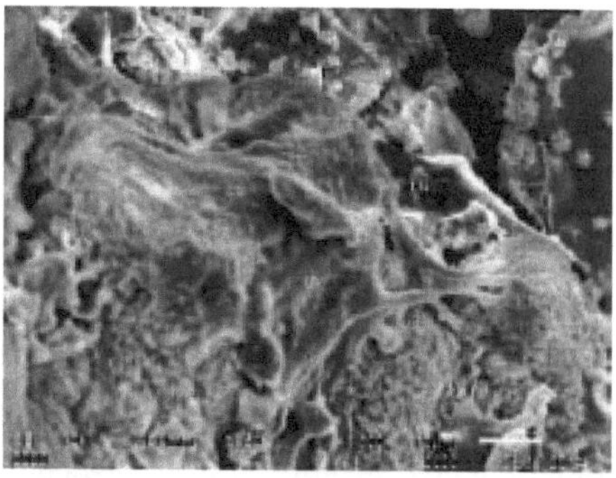

rBMSC seeded HASi on day 17 post-seeding showing cell sheet like structure (CSL) strongly anchored to scaffold by footpads (arrows)

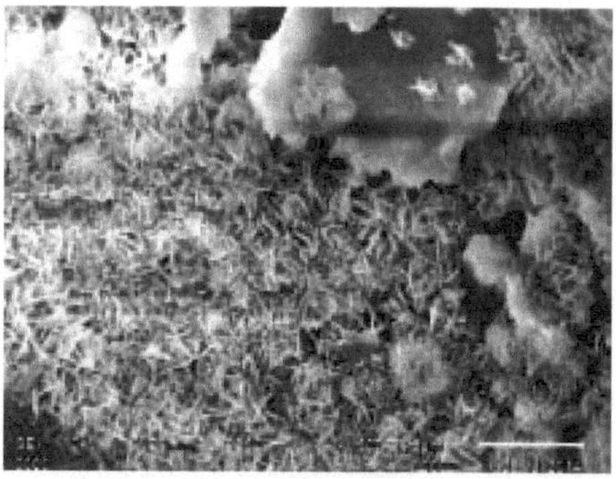

SEM analysis of rBMSC seeded HASi on day 17 post-seeding showing matrix deposition (arrows) over and around the attached cells

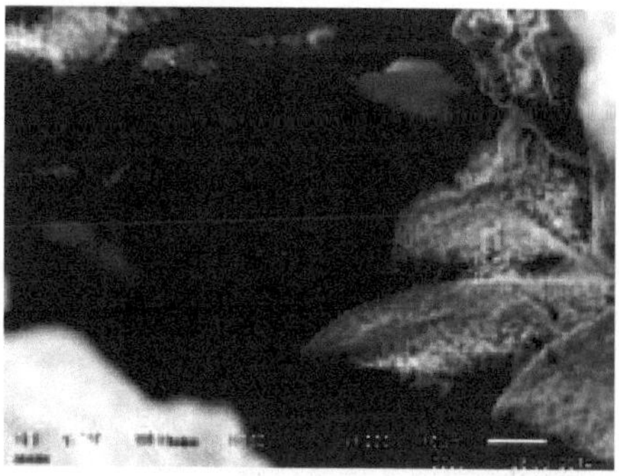

SEM analysis of rBMSC seeded HASi on day 17 post-seeding showing panoramic view of matrix deposition over attached cells

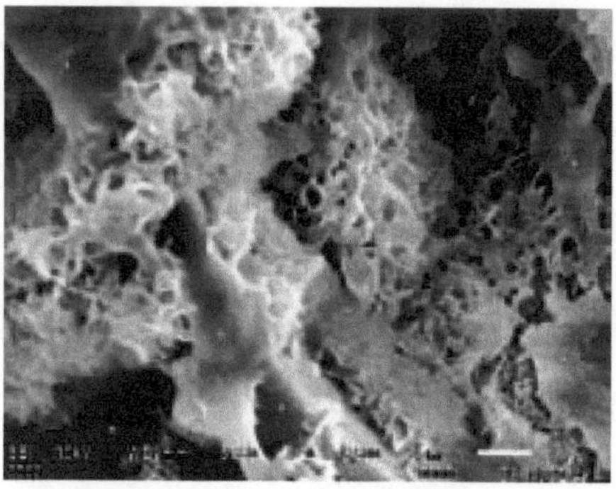

rBMSC seeded on HASi on day17 post-seeding showing calcium orthophosphate crystals (arrows) over attached cells (dots)

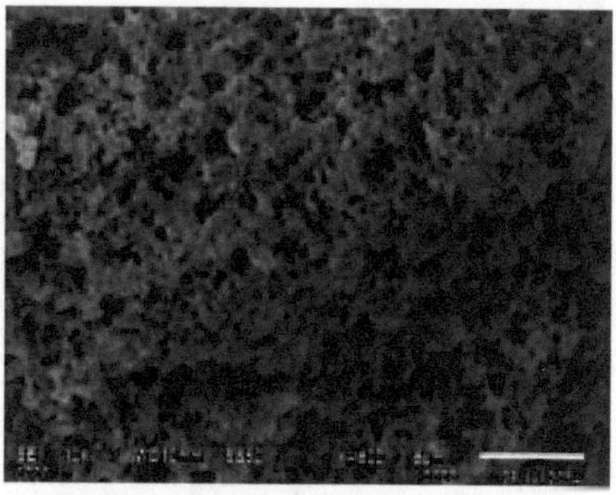

SEM analysis of the unseeded HASi after 17 days

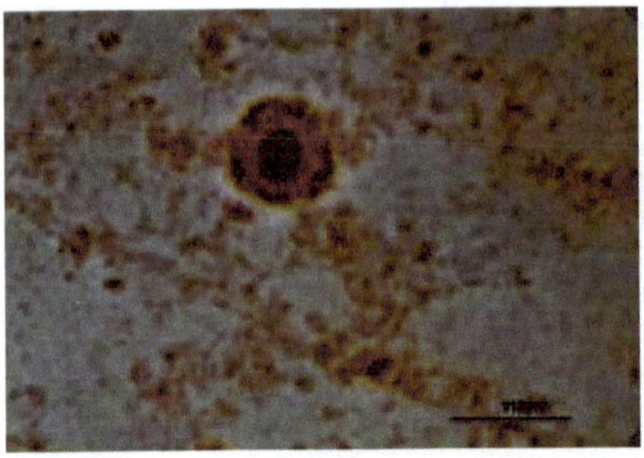

Micrograph of alizarin red stained calcium crystal trypsinized from day 17 post-seeding HASi showing positive intense red colour indicating of calcium

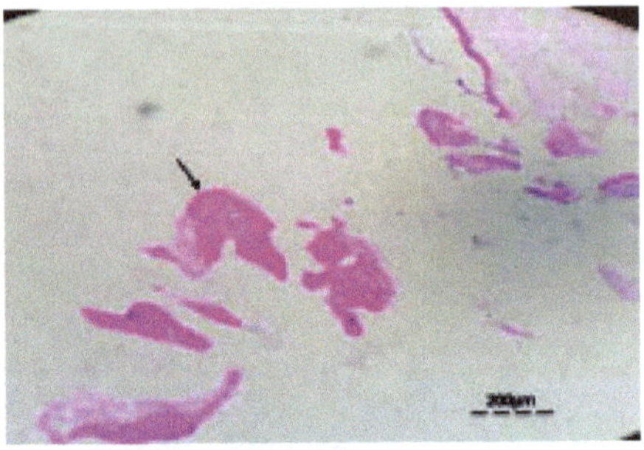

H & E stained sections of decalcified day 17 post-seeded HASi scaffold showing dark pink stained areas (arrows) indicating new bone formation

6

Implantation of MSC-Ceramic Construct for Repair of Critical Sized Bone Defect in Rabbit Model

Fracture healing is a complex process in which damaged bone restores its original architecture through a cascade of molecular and cellular events. The process of fracture healing is unique, in that it does not form a poorly organized replacement matrix, otherwise known as scar tissue, but rather regenerates the original matrix and retains its mechanical properties. Normal fracture and bone repair follows a known sequence of events includes: haematoma formation, inflammation, angiogenesis, osteogenesis, and bone remodeling.

For the repair of bone defects, a tissue engineering approach would be to combine cells capable of osteogenic (i.e. bone-forming) activity with an appropriate scaffolding material to stimulate bone regeneration and repair. An ideal tissue-engineered bone substitute should possess 3 elements: osteoprogenitor cells, osteoinductive factors, and an osteoconductive scaffold, and is considered as a potential substitute for autologous bone transplantation. Tissue engineering approaches have proven very effective in bone regeneration recently, and the successful repair of bone defects has been demonstrated in larger animals like canine, goat and sheep.

Stem cells from adult tissues are attractive materials for cell therapy, gene therapy, and tissue engineering. These cells generally have restricted lineage potential when compared to embryonic stem cells, and this may be advantageous in certain therapeutic applications. Till and McCulloch in 1961 describes the presence of hematopoietic progenitor cells in bone marrow. After this, the concept of MSCs is brought to light by Friedenstein and co-workers who demonstrated the osteogenic potential of BM cells by heterotrophic transplantation. Friedenstein and Owen called this cell an osteogenic stem cell or a BM stromal stem cell (Owen and Friedenstein, 1988). Although the pioneering work of Friedenstein and Owen is firmly established, the concept of non-hematopoietic stem cell came into light only after the publication of similar work by Pittenger *et al.* in

(1999). The term mesenchymal stem cells (MSCs) are first coined by Caplan (1991) as an alternative to "stromal" or "osteogenic" stem cell.

Mesenchymal stem cells are multipotential cells capable of proliferation and differentiation into osteogenic, chondrogenic and adipogenic lineages both *in vitro* and *in vivo*. MSCs are regarded as an excellent source of cells for bone tissue engineering because of their self replication and osteogenic differentiation capabilities. The use of autologous stem cells is not always desirable since the quality and/or quantity of such cells will be affected by old age, osteoporosis, and metabolic diseases. While allogenic BMSCs might be preferable to xenogenic ones, they are not always readily available. Further, allogenic MSCs have the potential for carrying disease, whereas the risk of such disease transmission might be minimized in genetically engineered animals that are specifically bred to serve as donors of BMSCs. Also the use of non- -autologous stem cells isolated from healthy donors offers a major advantage since these stem cells can be thoroughly tested and formulated into off-the-shelf medicine in advance. One of the attractive advantages of BMSCs as a source of cell transplantation is their low immunogenecity. Recently, several studies have reported that BMSCs may be immune-privileged cells that do not elicit immune responses due to an absence of their immunologically relevant cell surface markers.

In the last two decades, many of the bone substitute materials have been evaluated to replace the need for autologous or allogenic bone. Among them, the feasibility of bioactive ceramics, bioactive glasses, biological or synthetic polymers, and their composites for bone tissue engineering has been studied. Bioactive ceramics, namely HA, HA/TCP & bioactive glasses, have been used as scaffold for bone reconstruction for many years. They are termed 'bioactive' because they form an interfacial bond with tissues upon implantation and enhance bone tissue formation as a result of surface modification when exposed to interstitial fluids. Bioceramic provides scaffold to support the attachment and migration of newly formed bone cells into the osseous defect and also help in the formation of a vascular network through the newly formed bone. Bioceramic also acts as a carrier to deliver stem cells for osteogenesis and these bioactive inorganic materials are similar in composition to the mineral phase of bone that is of clinical interest.

Till now most of the xenogenic MSC transplantations for bone healing have been done from human to laboratory/large animal models of bone healing and between the two species of laboratory animals (rat & rabbit). The xenogenic transplantation of MSCs from small/large animal species to rabbit model of bone healing has not been attempted to the best of my knowledge. So, in this chapter, research work is planned with the following objectives: To develop and compare *in vitro* and *in vivo* system for induction of osteogenesis by different sources of BM-MSC construct for repairing critical size bone defect (CSD) in rabbit model and to evaluate the potentiality of cultured xenogenic mesenchymal stem cells for repairing radius critical-size bone defect (CSD) in rabbit model.

Experimental animals

The study is conducted on 36 male adult New Zealand White rabbits divided into six equal groups. They are kept in individual cages, fed a standard diet and allowed free mobilization during the study. The groups are compared as follows: The radial 15-mm segmental diaphyseal defect is filled with autogenous MSCs+ biphasic bio-ceramics (group A), allogenic MSCs + biphasic bioceramic (group B), ovine MSCs + biphasic bio-ceramic (group C), canine MSCs + biphasic bio-ceramic (group D), biphasic bio-ceramic (group E) and only empty bone defect (group E, control).

Collection, isolation, culture and expansion of bone marrow from rabbit, canine and sheep as described in previous chapter

In vivo osteogenesis of different stem cell (BMSCs) in Rabbit model

Anesthetic Protocol

The animals are anaesthetized using intramuscular injection of Xylazine (5mg/ kg) and Ketamine (50mg/kg) combination. For maintenance, Diazepam (5 mg/ ml) -Ketamine (50 mg/ ml) mixture is utilized at 1:1 ratio by intravenously.

Preparation of Critical sized bone defect (CSD) model

Surgery is performed under sterile condition. Right radius is exposed through medial approach. Mid shaft point of radius is determined by measuring the distance between radius head and styloid process. The 15mm full thickness critical sized defect (CSD) is created using hexa. For this matter, after skin incision and subcutaneous fascia undermining, the deep ante brachial fascia is incised between the extensor carpi radialis and pronator muscle proximally with paralleling the incision to the extensor carpi radialis in the distal portion of incision. After exposing the mid shaft of radius, CSD (15mm) is created and animals are treated based on their grouping. The CSD is not fixed by any internal fixation devices. Since the radius and ulna are adherent together tightly with interosseous membrane, adequate stability is achieved after osteotomy by leaving the ulna intact without any internal fixation of the radius. Following treatment implantation in respective groups, muscle and skin is sutured. The Critical size defect (CSD) of bone in each animal is filled with Biphasic TCP block alone or in combinations with other agents as listed.

Sub-group	Treatment	No. of animals
A	Autogenous MSCs + Biphasic TCP	6
B	Allogenic MSCs + Biphasic TCP	6
C	Ovine MSCs + Biphasic TCP	6
D	Canine MSCs + Biphasic TCP	6
E	Biphasic TCP	6
F	Bone defect (CSD) only	6

After implanting the Biphasic TCP bioceramic block alone or in combination with cultured autogenic, allogenic or xenogenic MSCs at the bone defect site, the muscles is apposed using 3-0 PGA and the skin is sutured with 1-0 nylon suture.

Tissue engineered construct

Inert, biodegradable, biphasic TCP bio-ceramic block (65% calcium hydroxyapatite, 35% tricalcium phosphate) with pore size 200-450 micrometer is taken and seeded with cultured bone marrow stem cell (BMSCs). Cells are seeded on biphasic TCP by centrifugal seeding. For this $4\text{-}5\times10^6$ cell suspension in 2 ml of growth media is added into a 2 ml eppendorf tube containing a scaffold. The solution is centrifuged at 30 g and 4^0 C for five minute intervals with mixing to resuspend the cell pallet between centrifugation intervals. The scaffolds are then incubated in the suspension of growth media at 37^0C and 5% CO2 in incubator for 12hrs and then used for implantation.

All the animals are kept in isolated cages and administered with broad spectrum antibiotic for 5 consecutive days. The analgesic is administered for 3 days. The wound is dressed until the complete healing of the incision is seen and sutures are removed. The animals are observed for the evidence of wound healing, radiographic bone healing postoperatively and they are euthanized for the study of gross morphology, histology, and scanning electron microscopy at 90th postoperative day.

Medio-lateral and anterio-posterior radiographs are taken immediately after implantation and subsequently on days 7, 15, 30, 60 and 90th postoperative day. Assessment of radiographic healing is done as per following table.

Radiographic grading scale for degree of new bone formation and critical sized defect (CSD) healing

Description	Score
– No change from immediate post-operative appearance	0
– A slight increase in radio density distinguished from the implant	1
– Recognizable increase in radio density of the implant with bridging of the cortex	2
– Callus formation with complete defect bridging	3
– Bridging at least one cortex with material of non-union radio density, easily incorporation of the implant suggested by obscurity of implant borders	4
– Defect bridged on both proximal and distal sides with bone of uniform radio density, cut ends of the cortex still visible, implant and new bone not easy to differentiate	5
- Same as grade 3, with at least one of four cortices obscured by new bone	6
– Defect bridged by uniform new bone, cut ends of cortex no longer distinguishable, implant no longer visible	7
– Complete union, complete new bone formation, complete cortex covered the defect, marrow cavity formed	8

Blood is collected before operation and at regular interval postoperatively for the estimation of different biochemical parameters viz. serum protein, serum glucose, serum alkaline phosphatase, serum calcium and serum phosphorus in each six groups using commercial available diagnostic kit.

The test bones are collected from the animals sacrificed on day 90 postoperatively and a 2.5 cm long piece of radius including the site of the defect and normal bone on both sides is cut using hexa saw. The bone segments are washed thoroughly with normal saline and fixed in 10% formalin for 48-72 hours. The segments are decalcified in Goodling and Stewart's fluid containing 15 ml formic acid, 5 ml formalin and 80 ml distilled water. Solution is stirred daily and changed once in 3 days. The sections are checked regularly for the status of decalcification. The completion of decalcification is assessed by flexibility, transparency and pin penetrability of the bone sections. The tissues are processed in a routine manner and 4 μ thick longitudinal sections are cut and stained with Hematoxylin and Eosin (H&E) as per the standard procedure. The assessment of histological bone healing is done by following table.

Histological grading scale for degree of healing

Scale	Description	Score
Quality of Union	No sign of fibrous or other union	0
	Fibrous union	1
	Fibro cartilage or cartilage union	2
	Mineralized cartilage and immature bone union	3
	Bone union	4

For scanning electron microscopy, the bone specimens for this study are collected from the test bone immediately after euthanizing the animals on day 90 postoperatively. Each specimen is consisted of both fracture healing site and adjacent bone. The samples are fixed in 2% glutaraldehyde phosphate buffer solution for 24-48 hours. After fixing in glutaraldehyde, two washings for 30 minutes each with phosphate buffer saline (pH 7.4) followed by distilled water is performed. Then the specimens are dehydrated in serial concentration of ethanol for 30 minutes. Thereafter, the specimens are dried with Hexamethyldisilazine (HMDS) for 20 minutes. Specimens are mounted on aluminum stubs using adhesive silicon tape. After that golden ion sputtering is done on Jeol ion sputter Model JFC 1600 at 7- 10 mA and 1-2 kv for 15 minutes. Finally, the specimens are observed under scanning electron microscope at appropriate acceleration voltage and the magnification range of the unit calibrated using colloidal latex particles of 1 μ size for the study of their different surfaces to identify the orientation and distribution of newly formed osseous tissue and distribution/ absorption of implant at the fracture site.

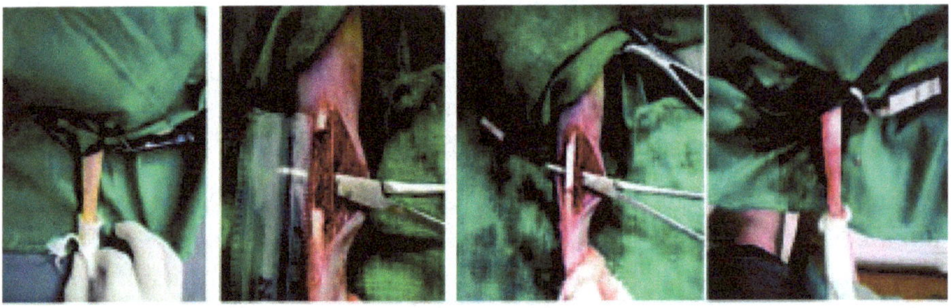

CSD= 15mm in Radius of NZW Rabbit

Radiographic evaluation is performed to record the acceptance or rejection of xenogenic MSCs, the initiation and progression of healing and bone formation at the critical size defect site. The mean score for all the parameters of radiographic evaluation of bone healing is found to be increasing with time in all the groups and differed significantly between groups at the corresponding time intervals. The overall total healing score for radiographic evaluation of bone healing shows significant variation in the healing among the groups at different time intervals and is suggestive different grades for healing. Due to overlapping of the radius by ulna in AP view, the radiographic evaluation is mostly involved analysis of mediolateral views of the radiographs.

Day 0: In mediolateral views of radiographs, the critical size defect is clearly visible with cut edges of the bone almost at the center of the radial diaphysis in all the animals of control group and this area is filled by bioceramic block with or without MSCs in comparison to the other groups. The defect site is completely filled with bioceramic block that looked relatively denser than the adjacent bone and this density is also considered while evaluating the bone healing.

Day 14: There is absolutely no change in the defect size in group F animals and it is same as on day 0. In case of group A and B, there is no evidence of callus formation but there is increase in the radiodensity of the block and slight periosteal reaction at the cut edges of the host bone. There is slight increase in the radio density of the bioceramic block in group C animals that could be easily distinguished by comparing it to day 0 radiographs. In group D animals there is no recognizable change in the implant area, but the host graft interface indicated some apposition between the two. In case of group C and D animals there is no graft rejection process, which is radiographically evident by absence of inflammatory response in and around the critical size defect area. The block is in the same position without change in its radiodensity in group E animals.

Day 30: Groups A and B animal's shows the new bone formation along with initiation of resorption of bioceramic block. The autologous transplanted group (A) shows more bridging of block with ulna bone compared to allogenic group (B). The latter group shows signs of union between the implant and host bone that is visible at the proximal and distal end of critical size defect. In case of ovine MSCs transplanted group (C), there is resorption of block with periosteal reaction that is evident clearly, which indicates the deposition of new bone into the bioceramic block. Canine MSCs transplanted group (D) also shows the initiation of osteoid deposition, which is visible by resorption of bioceramic block. In group E animals there is clear evidence of bridging of proximal end of the block with host bone. In group F animals, there is fibrous dense tissue appearance near the defect margins. The defect is clearly visible without any callus formation, as the fibrous tissue has not filled the entire defect.

Day 60: All the animals of group A shows increased new bone formation with periosteal reaction and increased resorption of block, which has led to loss of its shape. In allogenic group (group B), there is complete bridging of bioceramic block with the host bone at all the surface of contact which indicates the formation of new bone. In case of groups C and D there is complete bridging on both proximal and distal side with bone of uniform radio density, which indicated deposition of new osteoid bone into the bioceramic block by the osteoprogenitor cells. The bone formation is more or less similar in both C and D groups. In group E animals there is bridging of proximal end of the bioceramic block with host bone as it is evident on day 30. The control group (group F) is revealed appearance of fibrous dense tissue near the defect margins and has not filled the entire defect site.

Day 90: The autologous transplanted group (A) of animals shows excellent bone formation, which is evident radiographically by resorption of bioceramic block and bridging of block completely with the host bone, which has lost its shape completely. In allogenic transplanted group (B) of animals also shows good bone formation, which is evident radiographically by bridging of bioceramic block completely with the host bone at all the surface of contact. At this stage both the xenogenic transplanted groups (C and D), shows better bone formation compared to control (group F) and biphasic tricalcium phosphate group (E), but there is less bone formation in comparison to autologous and allogenic groups (A and B). The radiograph of control group (F) animals at this stage shows more fibrous tissue at the cut ends of radius bone compared to day 60, but there is no union of the ends by any of the structure. Group E animal's shows bridging of proximal end of block with host bone.

On the basis of radiographic observation, it can be conclude that application of xenogenic BM-MSCs of canine and ovine origin, seeded with bioceramic block induces faster bone formation without immunological rejection and inflammatory reaction in critical size defects (CSDs) compared to control and BCP block alone. However the results are inferior in comparison to autologous and allogenic BMSCs transplanted groups.

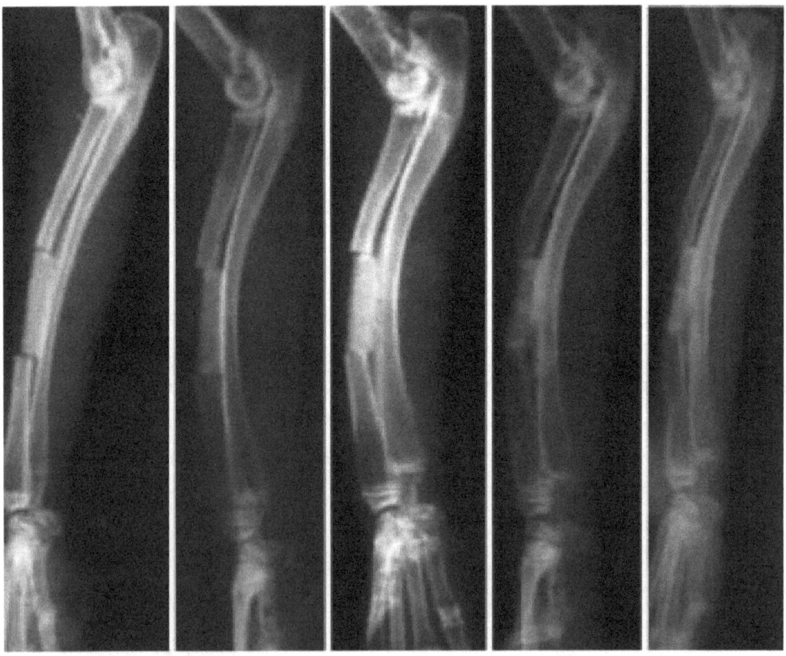

Day 0 Day 14 Day 30 Day 60 Day 90

Sequential medio-lateral radiographs of group A

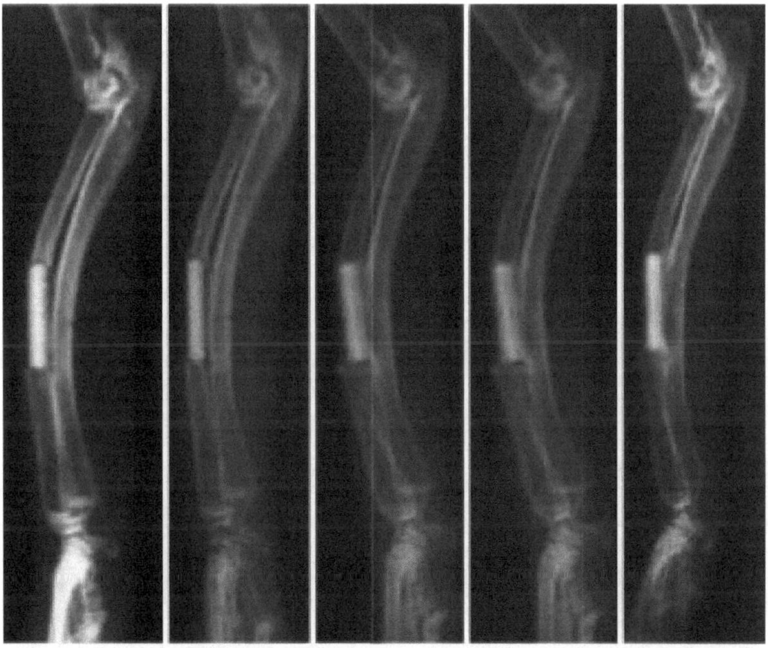

Day 0 Day 14 Day 30 Day 60 Day 90

Sequential medio-lateral radiographs of group B

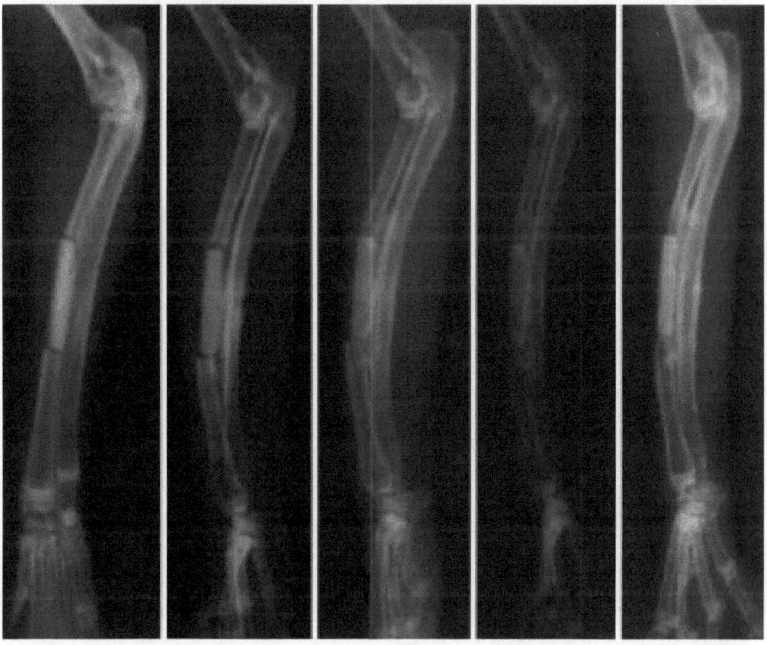

Day 0 Day 14 Day 30 Day 60 Day 90

Sequential medio-lateral radiographs of group C

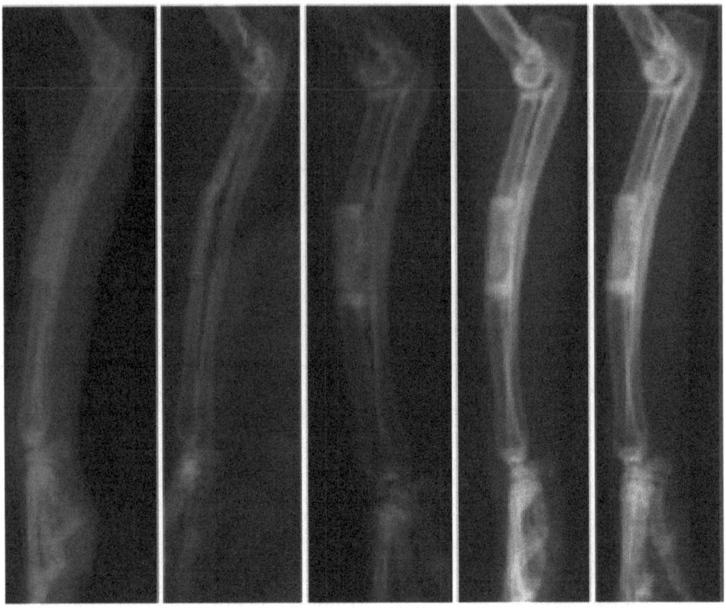

Day 0 Day 14 Day 30 Day 60 Day 90

Sequential medio-lateral radiographs of group D

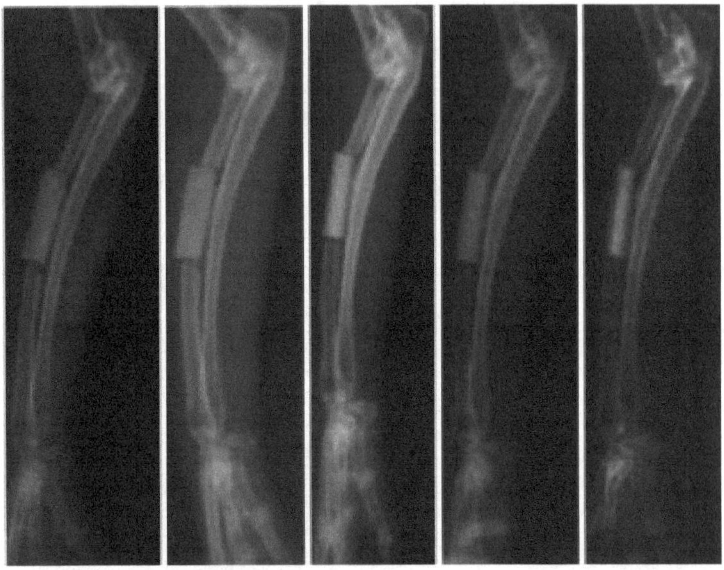

Day 0 Day 14 Day 30 Day 60 Day 90

Sequential medio-lateral radiographs of group E

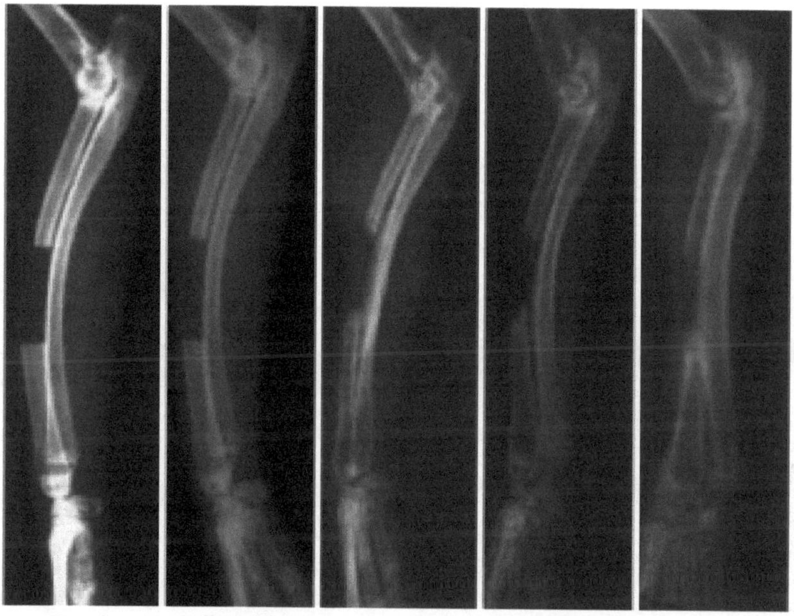

Day 0 Day 14 Day 30 Day 60 Day 90

Sequential medio-lateral radiographs of group F

The mean values for different biochemical parameters in various groups are shown in below table. There is no significant difference is observed except mild increase in ALP level is noticed in all the groups.

The mean ± S.E. values for different biochemical parameters

Sl no.	Parameters	Gr- 1	Gr- 2	Gr- 3	Gr- 4	Gr- 5	Gr- 6
1	Calcium (mg/dl)	10.64 ±1.20	9.61 ±0.91	10.57 ±0.73	10.14 ±0.62	10. 10 ±1.01	11.41 ±0.91
2	Phosphorus (mg/dl)	5. 38 ±0.65	4. 37 ±0.65	4.93 ±0.50	5.22 ±0.42	5. 51 ±0.44	5. 26 ±0.62
3	Total protein (g/dl)	6.69 ±1.08	5. 57 ±0.59	6. 63 ±1.04	6. 60 ±0.45	6. 28 ±0.88	6. 61 ±0.69
4	Glucose (mg/dl)	82. 03 ±8.33	63. 30 ±6.72	70.96 ±8.97	97. 33 ±16.43	73. 66 ±12.87	78.02 ±9.66
5	ALP (KAU)	17. 08 ±0.43	16. 69 ±1.02	17. 01 ±0.90	19. 65 ±1.64	16. 45 ±1.39	17.15 ±1.40

Radiographic score between different groups in different time interval

Group	Day 0	Day 14	Day 30	Day60	Day 90	Total
Group A	0±0.00	1.2±0.09	2.5±0.34	3.8±0.43	4.5±0.45	12.00±0.32
Group B	0±0.00	0.9±0.45	1.9±0.22	3.4±0.23	4.02±0.05	10.22±0.23
Group C	0±0.00	0.6±0.78	2.7±0.67	2.9±0.57	3.98±0.78	10.18±0.70
Group D	0±0.00	0.7±0.87	2.9±0.56	3.5±0.23	4..1±0.77	11.20±0.60
Group E	0±0.00	0.3±0.12	1.45±0.66	2.1±0.45	2.2±0.12	06.05±0.33
Group F	0±0.00	0±0.00	0.2±0.22	0.3±0.12	0.44±0.89	0.94±0.24

Histological score between different groups at 90th day

Implanted group Average ± Standard Deviation	Histological Score
Group A	3.0±0.23
Group B	2.7±0.65
Group C	1.9±0.63
Group D	2.2±0.32
Group E	1.5±0.23
Group F	0.2±0.01

Histological observation

After euthanasia on 90th day, the sample are collected from defect sites approximately 2 mm proximal and 2 mm distal to the defect in a way the healing as well as the connection between new formed bone and old bone can be observed in a shot. After decalcification, the tissues are processed in a routine manner and 4 μ thick longitudinal sections are cut and stain with Hematoxylin and Eosin (H&E) for histological evaluation.

Group A: In this group, the periosteum is normal and completely surrounded the ceramic block. Defect is completely filled with immature and mature bone trabeculae, with the trabeculae being more immature at the centre compared to periphery of the ceramic block. Most of the scaffolds are substituted by newly formed bone with residual scaffold material that is visible in all TCP treated defects at 12 weeks postoperatively. The stain tissue section shows varying colors of pink with mineralized matrix seen as bright pink and the cell nuclei stain dark purple. The granular dense colour material in-between the trabecular structure indicates the remnant of graft material, which is less in this group and at higher magnification, osteoblastic lineage is clearly observed around the new bone with many osteocytes.

Group B: Newly formed bone is observed in all the animals of this group. The normal periosteum is completely surrounded the ceramic block. The formation of bone trabecular is observed throughout the bioceramic graft, which is more mature at the junction compared to centre of the graft. The group shows substitution of most of the scaffolds by new bone with minimal residual scaffold. At the junction of the graft material there is higher amount of mature bone formation. The gap between the trabecular bones is minimal. Lamellar bone formation is seen into porous HA/TCP implant at higher magnification.

Group C: The block is surrounded by the normal periosteum in all the animals. The formation of bone trabeculae is observed throughout the bioceramic graft with mature type confined to junction of the graft. The residual transplant has minimal volume which indicates the amount of the original HA/TCP scaffold that has been resorbed. On H& E stain examination, the bone stain pink, ceramic has a shadowy white appearance; loose connective tissue stain light pink and cells stain dark purple. There are no signs of inflammatory reaction to the scaffold in any of the animals in this group.

Group D: The normal periosteum is completely surrounded by the ceramic block. The formation of bone trabecular is observed throughout the bioceramic graft, which is more mature at the junction and periphery of the graft compared to central area. The gap between the trabeculae is minimal and is occupied by residual granular material. At the junction of graft, the lamellar bone formation is seen at higher magnification along with proliferating osteoprogenitor cells. There are no signs of any inflammatory reaction to the scaffold in any of the animals in this group.

Group E: The periosteal reaction surrounding the block is minimal in this group. The formation of immature bone trabecular is observed throughout the bioceramic implanted area. The gap between the trabeculae is comparatively more and is occupied by residual granular material. There are no mature bone trabeculae at the junction or periphery of the block area. Most of the area of the block is filled with fibrous connective tissue which stain light pink colour throughout the graft. No phagocytes are observed in the evaluated sections, which indicates HA/TCP ceramics are highly biocompatible.

Group F: There is no evidence of bone formation in any of the animals at the defect site. There is proliferation of dense fibro vascular connective tissue and inflammatory reaction at the junction of the defect. The entire gap is filled with fibro vascular tissue.

Scanning Electron Microscopic (SEM) Observations

For SEM examination, the bone specimens are collected on day 90 after sacrifice of the experimental animals. The scanning is done at the junction of healing bone defect with block and the adjacent normal bone to study status of bone formation, type of tissue involved inside the bioceramic block, the fate of hydroxyapatite and tricalcium phosphate, vascularity and extent of extracellular bone matrix, and the type of osseous tissue formed.

Group A: A close contact without intervening soft tissue is seen between bone and the graft. The osseous tissue is predominantly seen at the junction of graft and host bone. There is presence of bone inside macropores of hydroxyapatite and tricalcium phosphate throughout surface of the block. By using SEM the micropores structure in HA/TCP block can be visualized demonstrating a pore size of a 8.5 microns in diameter. The bone inside macropores reaching into the outer micropores of scaffolds is seen. Evaluation of the contents of micropores inside the block material is not possible using SEM. The micron-sized micropores inside the block are infiltrated by bony tissue and the collagen fibrils demonstrated a direct bone-to-material contact.

Group B: There is strong bridging of bioceramic block with the host bone by mature osseous bony structure. The bone formation is seen throughout the surface of graft inside the micro pores. The bone inside macropores reaching into the outer micropores of scaffolds is seen. Collagen fibrils are arranged in irregular manner and their density is more. Comparatively the scaffold material is lower, with higher bone formation in this group.

Group C: The bioceramic block is in close contact with the host bone by newly formed osseous tissue. The entire micropores of the bioceramic block are filled with bony structure. The bone inside macropores reaching into the outer micropores of scaffolds is seen and found denser. The collagen fibrils that connect newly formed bone with the scaffold are more in number. The resorption of hydroxyapatite and tricalcium phosphate is seen, which is evident by reduction in the volume of scaffold that is filled by newly formed bone.

Group D: In all the animals of this group, the block is strongly bound to host bone by newly formed osseous tissue. The entire micropores of the bioceramic block are completely filled with bony structure and there is no visible space between the microstructure inside the graft. The collagen fibrils are densely packed between the bone the graft material which indicates denser bone formation. The HA/TCP is relatively less in volume and that volume is replaced by newly formed bone.

Group E: In this group of animals the bridging of bioceramic graft with host bone is evident, but it is not strong unlike other groups. The surface of the block reveals more of the graft material as such which reveals less resorption of the hydroxyapatite and tricalcium phosphate in this group. Inside the micropores, the new bone formation is noticed but the quantity is less. The collagen, which bridges the newly formed bone with the scaffold, is relatively less.

Group F: In this group of animals, there is no formation of bone at the entire length of the defect. The defect is filled with fibrous like structure. The cut edges of bone are having some projection. Evaluation of the contents inside the projected material is not possible by using SEM.

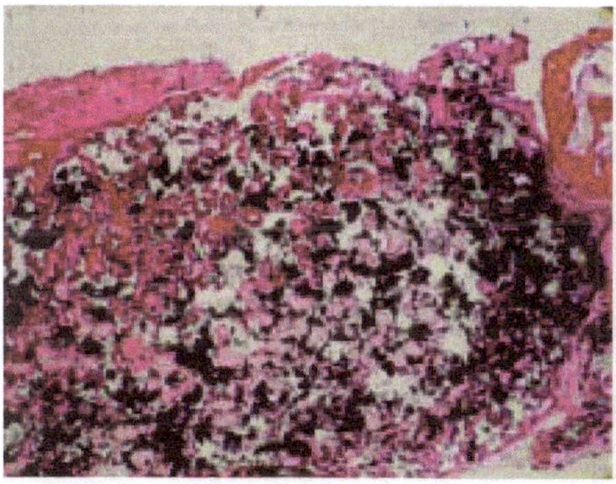

Group-A

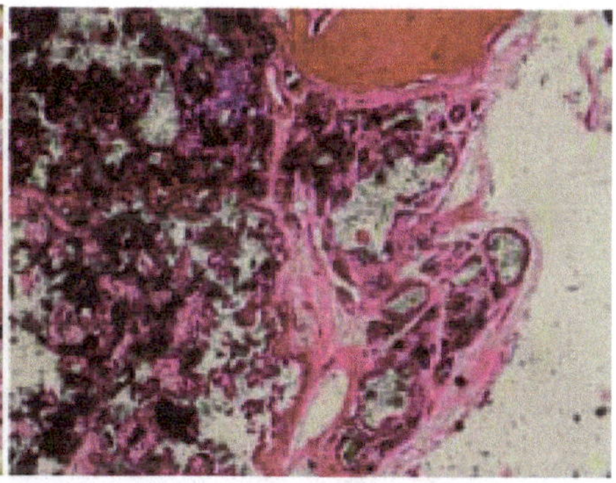

Group-A

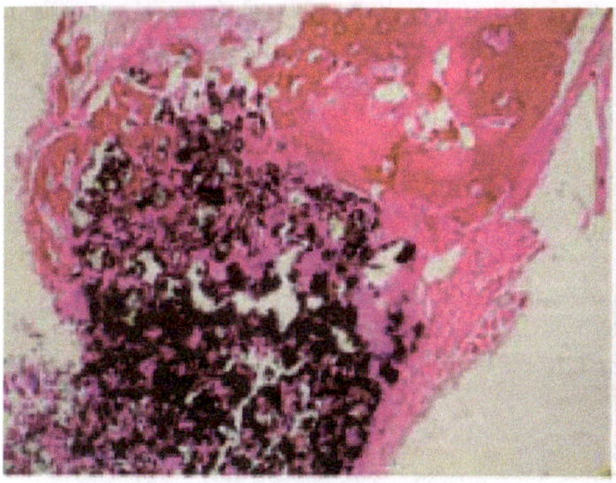

Group-B

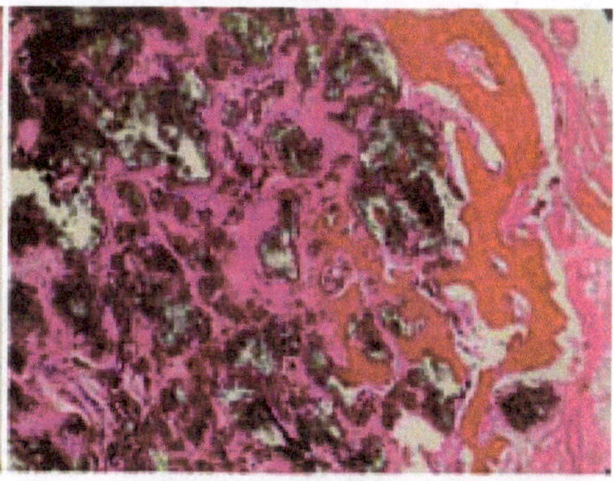

Group-B

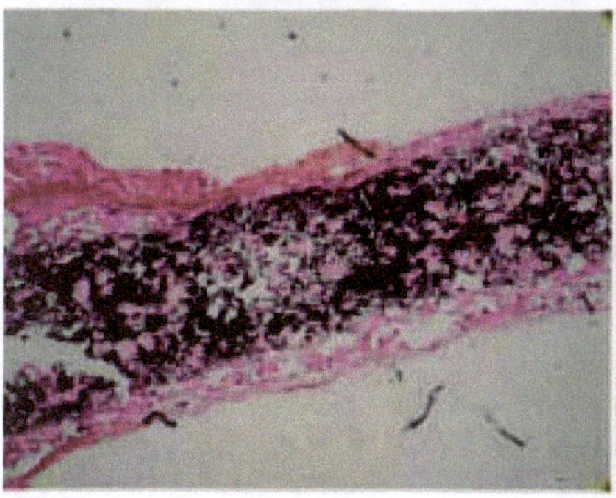

Group-C

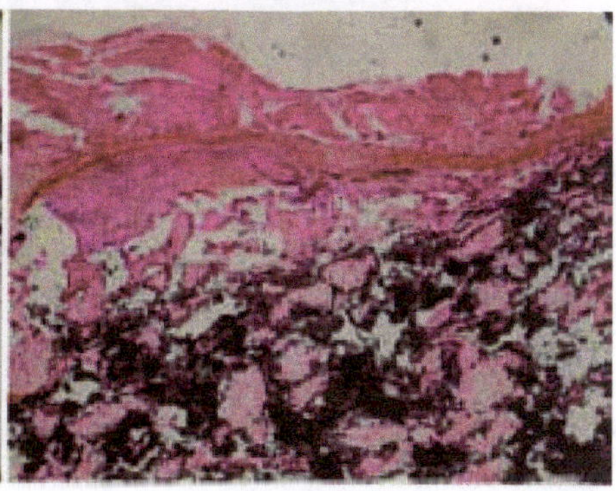

Group-C

Histopathological observations

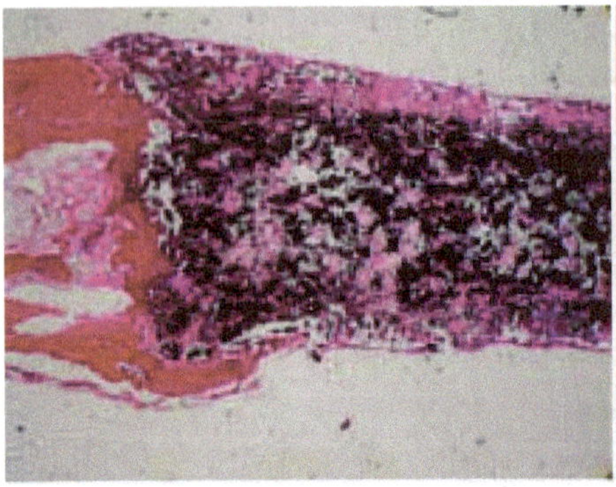

Group-D

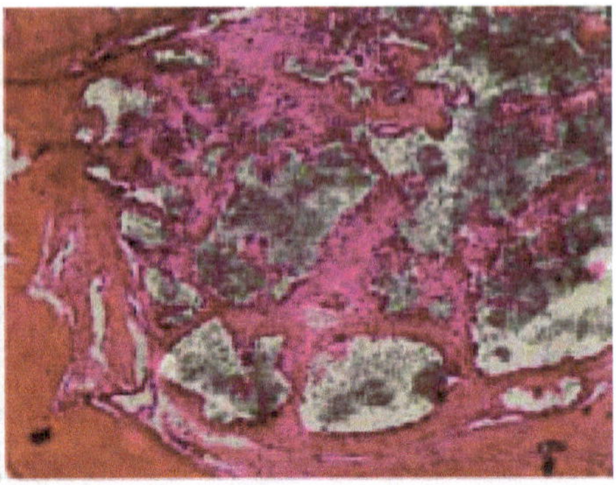

Group-D

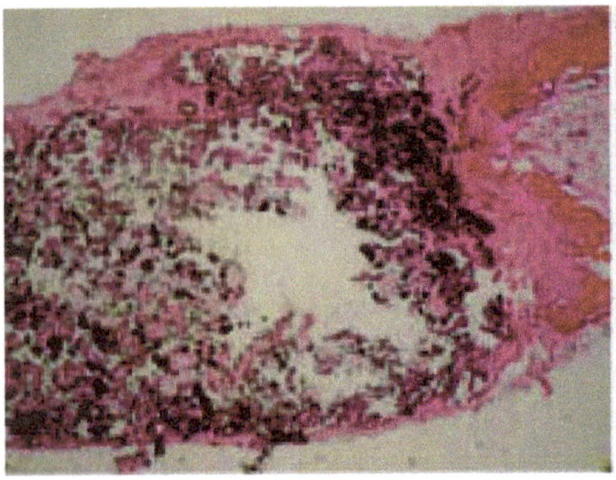

Group-E

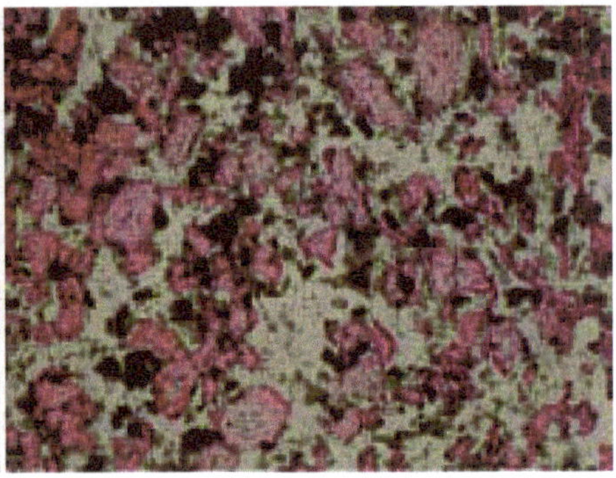

Group-E

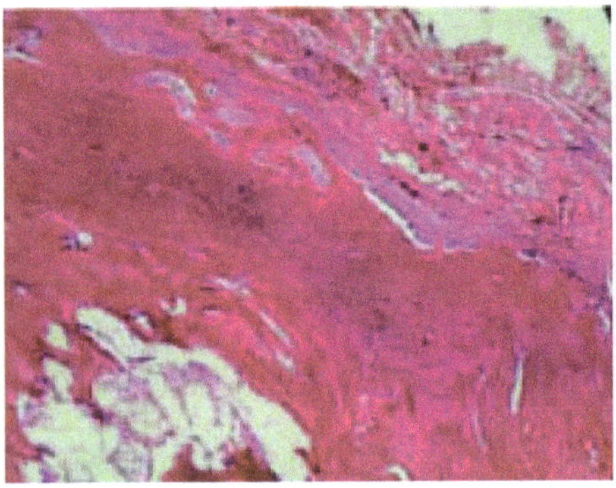

Group-F

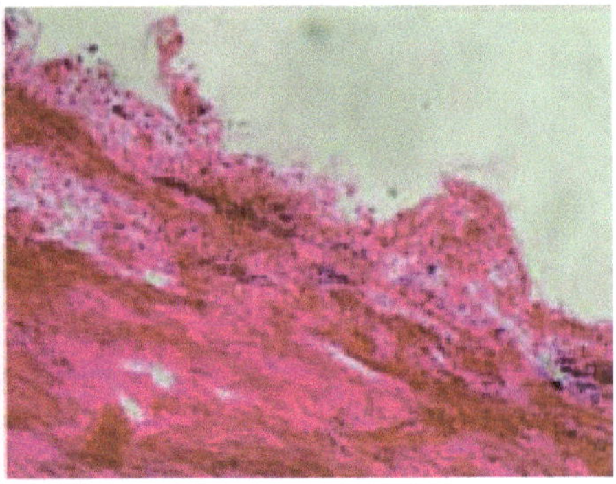

Group-F

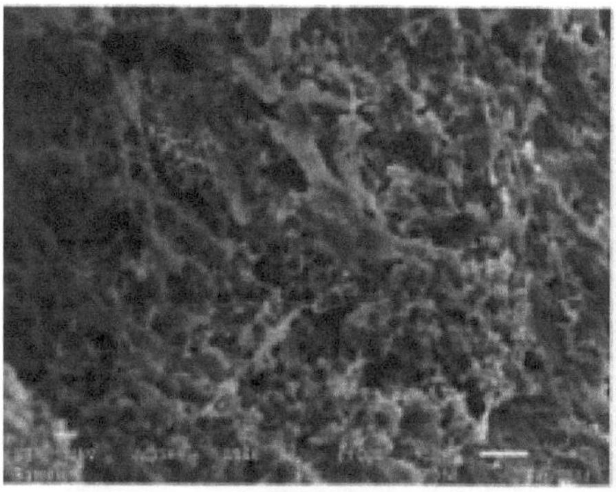

Group-A

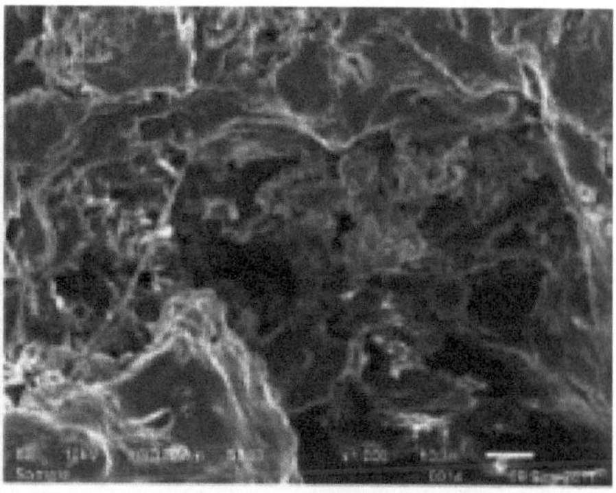

Group-B

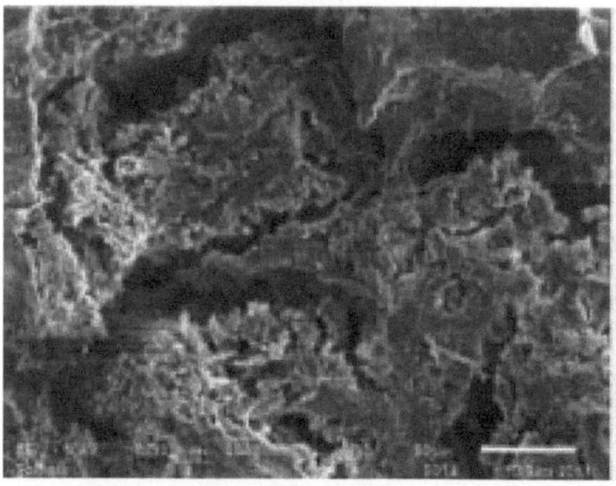

Group-C

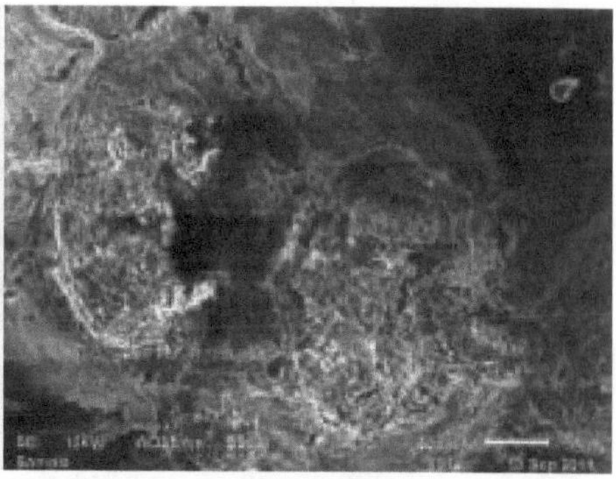

Group-D

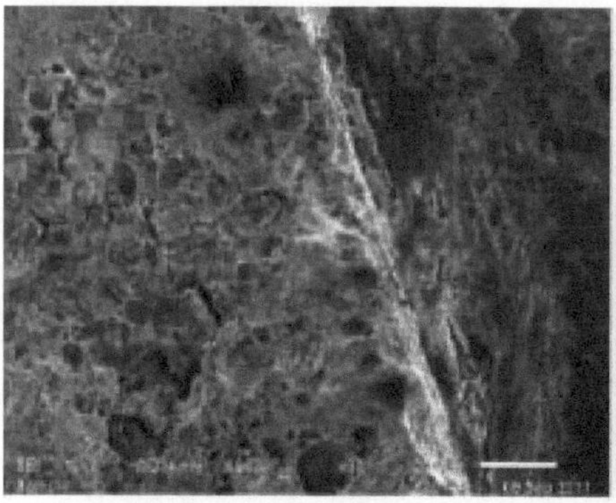

Group-E

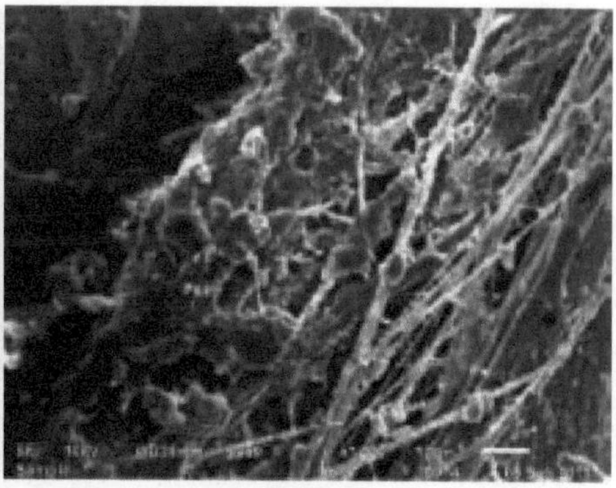

Group-F

Scanning electron microscopic (SEM) observations

7

Mesenchymal Stem Cells Seeded Bioceramic Construct for Bone Regeneration in Large Critical-size Bone Defect in Rabbit

Despite the benefits that minimally invasive surgery and osteosynthesis have brought to fracture management and bone healing, there are still many circumstances where bone healing remains challenging. Large bone defects are serious complications that are most commonly caused by extensive trauma, tumour, infection, or congenital musculoskeletal disorders. In nonunion cases repairing of bone defects with composite biomaterials as defect filler can promote bone regeneration. Currently, the gold standard for bone regeneration is use of autogenous bone graft. In order to avoid morbidity at the donor site or if large amount of autogenous bone is needed, bone substitution materials can be used.

Bone substitution materials can be combined with cells such as mesenchymal stem cells (MSCs) to increase bone formation. Bone-marrow derived mesenchymal stem cells (BMSCs) represent an attractive cell population for tissue regeneration. Bone marrow stem cells are pluripotent cells that have been used to facilitate bone repair because of their capability of differentiating into osteoblasts. Several studies on the regeneration of bone have shown that cultured BMSCs, seeded on different bioabsorbable implants are able to induce bone formation *in vivo* and lead to improved healing of critical-size defects.

Calcium phosphate bone substitutes such as hydroxyapatite (HA) and tricalcium phosphate (TCP) are currently used for bone substitution in many different clinical applications such as repair of bone defects after trauma or tumour and bone augmentation in spinal arthrodesis. Although these bone substitutes are osteoconductive, they often lack the osteogenecity needed to support bone healing in large defects and are slowly degraded in the body. Studies have shown that coating of hydroxyapatite with a calcium silicate layer could encourage cell proliferation and osteogenic differentiation of human bone marrow-derived stromal cells. Silica-calcium phosphate composite in comparison to calcium phosphate-rich biomaterials has a faster resorption rate owing to greater dissolution of Si ions.

The use of several growth factors have been studied in bone repair and these factors are known to play a role in differentiation of mesenchymal progenitor cells specific lineages like endothelial cells or osteoblasts. Bone morphogenetic protein-2 (BMP-2) has been shown to accelerate bone healing in humans and animal models. BMP-2 acts by osteoinduction and is involved in the differentiation of mesenchymal progenitor cells into osteoblasts. The addition of recombinant human BMP (rhBMP-2) to a self-cross linkable cellulose hydrogels/biphasic calcium phosphate granules construct promotes bone regeneration in a critical-size segmental defect model of non-union in dogs. It is also reported that protein, insulin-like growth factor (IGF-1) stimulates direct migration of human mesenchymal progenitor cells (MPC) and contributes to the recruitment of MPC in bone formation and bone healing.

Transplantation of human mesenchymal stem cells in a non-autogenous setting for bone regeneration in a rabbit critical-size defect (15mm) has been reported, but the regeneration potential of autogenous MSC with or without growth factors beyond standard critical-size defect is not reported. So, in this chapter, the potential of cultured autogenic rabbit bone marrow derived mesenchymal stem cells (rBMSC) seeded in a triphasic composite bio-scaffold (namely HASi) to generate new bone formation in an extensively large (30mm) segmental diaphyseal bone defect in rabbit model with or without growth factors rhBMP-2 and IGF-1 is described.

Experimental design

The study is conducted on 30 female adult New Zealand White rabbits divided into five equal groups. The groups are compare as follows: The radial 30-mm segmental diaphyseal defect is fill with a HASi scaffold only (group B); HASi scaffold seeded with autogenous rBMSC (group C); HASi scaffold seeded with autogenous rBMSC along with rhBMP-2 (group D) and HASi scaffold seeded with autogenous rBMSC along with IGF-1 (group E). An empty defect serves as the control group (group A).

A triphasic composite bio-scaffold namely HASi with elements in the following percentage: calcium-66.36%, Phosphorus- 25.35%, Silicon- 8.29% and porosity of 50 – 500 μm is used as ceramic bloc. Each HASi block is of 30 mm long and 5 mm in diameter are produced in an emulsion process.

Isolation and culture of rBMSC is performed as describe in earlier chapter. The rBMSCs at passage 3 are used for this experiment.

The HASi bioscaffold are incubated at 4^{0}C in fibronectin soln diluted in PBS for 24 h. Five million rBMSC are re-suspended in 4 ml of culture medium and transferred into a 5 ml tube. The HASi blocks are placed into the medium containing the cells. After 1.5 h of continuous spinning at 37^{0}C, the ceramic blocks are placed into a 6-well plate. The medium containing the cells is centrifuged twice, and the resulting cell pellet is re-suspended in culture medium and applied to the ceramic blocks. This MSC seeded ceramic scaffold is used in group C. Tissue engineered bone construct for group D is consisted of seeded HASi scaffold along with rhBMP-2 suspended in DMEM, placed at the implant site, whereas, in group E, seeded HASi scaffold along with IGF-1 suspended in DMEM placed at the implant site. In group B, only HASi block/scaffold is used at the implant site.

Under general anesthesia with Xylazine hydrochloride and Ketamine hydrochloride and strict surgical asepsis, a unilaterally critical-size bone defects are created in the radial diaphysis. A 4 cm super medial incision over the radius is given, soft tissue is dissected and the bone exposed by gentle retraction of the muscles. A Hohmann retractor is placed between ulna and radius to protect the ulna. A 30 mm segmental osteo-periosteal diaphyseal defect is created with an oscillating bone saw that is continuously cooled by irrigation with 0.9% sterile cold saline solution. The periosteum is removed with the bone and 5mm of periosteum is stripped from each side of the remaining radius. The bone gap is irrigated with sterile physiological saline solution and ceramic block (or nothing) fitted into the gap as per treatment protocol for different groups. Muscles, fascia and skin are separately closed over the defect with 4-0 resorbable sutures. A wooden splint with bandage is applied on the test bone for one week.

Postoperatively, broad spectrum antibiotic is administered intramuscularly for five days. Analgesic is given for the first 3 postoperative days. After 90 days of experiment, the animals are sacrificed.

Craniocaudal and mediolateral radiographic view of each ostectomy site is assessed immediately after surgery to monitor the position of the implants, and on 7, 15, 30, 45, 60 and 90 days postoperatively to assess bone formation and bone union with the host bone at both proximal and distal junctions.

Microcomputed tomography (μCT) technique is used for evaluation of three dimensional trabecular new bone formation in different treatment groups. On day 90 after implantation, the constructs are explanted after euthanizing the animals, preserving both proximal and distal interfaces. Images are acquired under 70keV voltage with a constant 114 μA current.

On day 90 post-implantation, the animals are sacrificed. The test bone sections throughout the length of the defect are collected from the site of surgical implant and washed thoroughly with sterile normal saline solution. Fixation is done in 10% formalin. The bone sections are subjected to decalcification in Goodling and Stewart solution. The decalcified bone sections are stained by H & E and Masson's trichrome stain. The sections are examined using a light microscope under different magnification.

Result

Weight bearing on the operated limb is mild to moderate from day 3 after surgery in all groups except group A. Complete weight bearing is seen after removal of wooden splint in all animals of groups B, C, D and E on day 7 after surgery. In the control group the animals do not bear weight normally throughout the experiment period. No animal of this group A is survived on day 90 due to complete lameness. The implanted biomaterials do not cause any apparent signs of irritation or infection and cutaneous wound healing is uneventful.

The radiographic analysis is done based on mediolateral view as there is overlapping of the radius by ulna in craniocaudal view. In control group (A), on day 30, the osteotomy line at defect site become invisible marking the progress of bone repair near this cut end. On day 45, a slight increase in radio-opacity is seen near this defect, marking the beginning of callus formation. On day 60, the area of radio-opacity is seen to be spread a little more and the defect remaining unbridged. No animal of control group is survived on day 90 as there is complete fracture of remaining ulna causes complete lameness and unable to stand or walk. In group B, mild resorption of the construct is started on day 45 and on day 60, the resorption is moderate. There is gap between the construct and the cut ends of host bone till day 60 but there is increased bone density at the junction of construct with the ulna on day 90. There is no evidence of bridging at either proximal or distal end of ceramic block with the host bone. Osteogenic process is very negligible. In group C, bridging of the bone and construct at proximal end is seen from day 30 onwards. On day 60, there is close attachment of the construct with the adjacent ulna and bridging between composite construct and cut end of the host bone. On day 90, good amount of new bone formation is noticed and the construct also underwent moderate resorption by this time. In group D, bridging between host bone and implant in both proximal and distal interfaces is evident at day 30. On day 45, there is close union between composite scaffold and the adjacent ulna. On day 60, a major portion of the construct is underwent resorption and the boundary between implant and normal bone disappear, which indicates that the implant has been replaced by early new bone. This is more pronounced on day 90. In group E, there is bony union between scaffold and ulna on day 45, whereas, bridging of both the proximal and distal defect ends with the host bone is seen on day 60. Moderate resorption of construct and bridging with adjacent ulna is more evident on day 90.

Micro computed tomography assessment is able to distinguish between the three phases present inside the defects: newly formed bone, remaining triphasic bioceramic block and non-mineralized tissues. The transverse and longitudinal sections reveal the unbridged cut ends of the host radius and there is no osteogenic reaction in-between radius and adjacent ulna in any of the animal group A. In other groups, newly formed trabecular bone at the defect site in radius bone is seen. The HASi component in defect site is almost intact in group B, whereas it is in the process of resorption in groups C, D and E. In group C, signs of osteogenesis and process of remodeling are observed. In group D, transverse and longitudinal bone sections show the establishment of periosteal continuity in between the cut ends of old host bone and continuation of medullary cavity at the defect site. Newly formed trabecular bone is under remodeling process in groups D and E.

Histopathological sections in control group (A), majority of the defect area are occupied by fibrous tissue. In group B, very little new woven bone formation, which is discontinuous in nature, is seen at the junction of scaffold and cut ends of the host bone. The scaffold is in the process of resorption and localized regions of new bone formation are seen as dispersed islands. In group C, new woven bone formation at the junction of scaffold and cut ends of host bone and osteochondral union between the ulna and scaffold is seen. There is invasion of periosteum from the adjacent ulna into the defect area. The scaffold is under active resorption and replaced by newly formed woven bone at some places. In group D, abundant new dense bone tissue formation and close bony union of scaffold with the host bone at both cut ends as well as with the adjacent ulna is seen. Scaffold is under active resorption and many places it is replaced by newly formed woven bone. Increased vascularisation near the junction between scaffold and the adjacent ulna is seen. Marrow formation is also evident in more than half of the implant area indicative of remodeling. Osteogenesis process is of intramembraneous type without any intermediate cartilage formation. Masson's trichrome staining is revealed close association of newly formed bone in the defect area with the host bone represented by more areas of mineralization and new osteoid tissue. In group E, osteochondral union is seen between the scaffold and cut ends of host bone as well as with the ulna. Three -fourth of the scaffold has undergone cartilaginous transition and areas of new bone formation are evident.

In this study since the defect size is too large, uses a custom designed external splint which is maintained for 7 days. No significant bone formation and consolidation of the defect is achieved in any animal in which the defect is left untreated -control group. Since the purpose of this study is to investigate the influence of MSC with or without growth proteins; empty scaffolds are used as an additional control group. In the bioceramic group (B) there is no evidence of bridging at either proximal or distal end of ceramic block with the host bone on day 90 post implantation. Osteogenic process is very negligible. In a further control group, a combination of autogenous MSC and HASi is transplanted into the defect area. In these animals, increased bone formation is found compared with HASi alone. Radiological, μCT and histological analysis shows bony union between the scaffold and cut ends of the host bone as well as with the adjacent ulna. Mesenchymal stem cells are known to have the ability to undergo osteogenic differentiation under suitable conditions. Their proliferation and differentiation capacity may be enhanced by exposing them to growth factors. Growth factors are protein signaling agents that act locality to stimulate formation and proliferation of osteoblasts and thereby promote bone healing. The rhBMP-2-treated constructs in group D encourages the formation of abundant bone tissue bridging both proximal and distal interfaces as well as with adjacent ulna as early as eight weeks after surgery. On day 90 after surgery, μCT and histopathological analysis shows newly formed bony tissue within the implantation site. Periosteal continuity is complete at the defect site with host bone. Histological and μCT analysis in group E reveal that there is osteochondral union and cartilaginous transition between implant and host bone at defect site as well as with the adjacent ulna. The findings of this study shows that *in vitro* seeding of autogenous rBMSC on HASi hasten the osteoconductive properties of scaffold and can be alternative to autogenous bone graft in the treatment of large bone defects and non-union. Addition of growth proteins particularly rhBMP-2 to autogenous MSC seeded HASi bioceramic construct can accelerate bone regeneration.

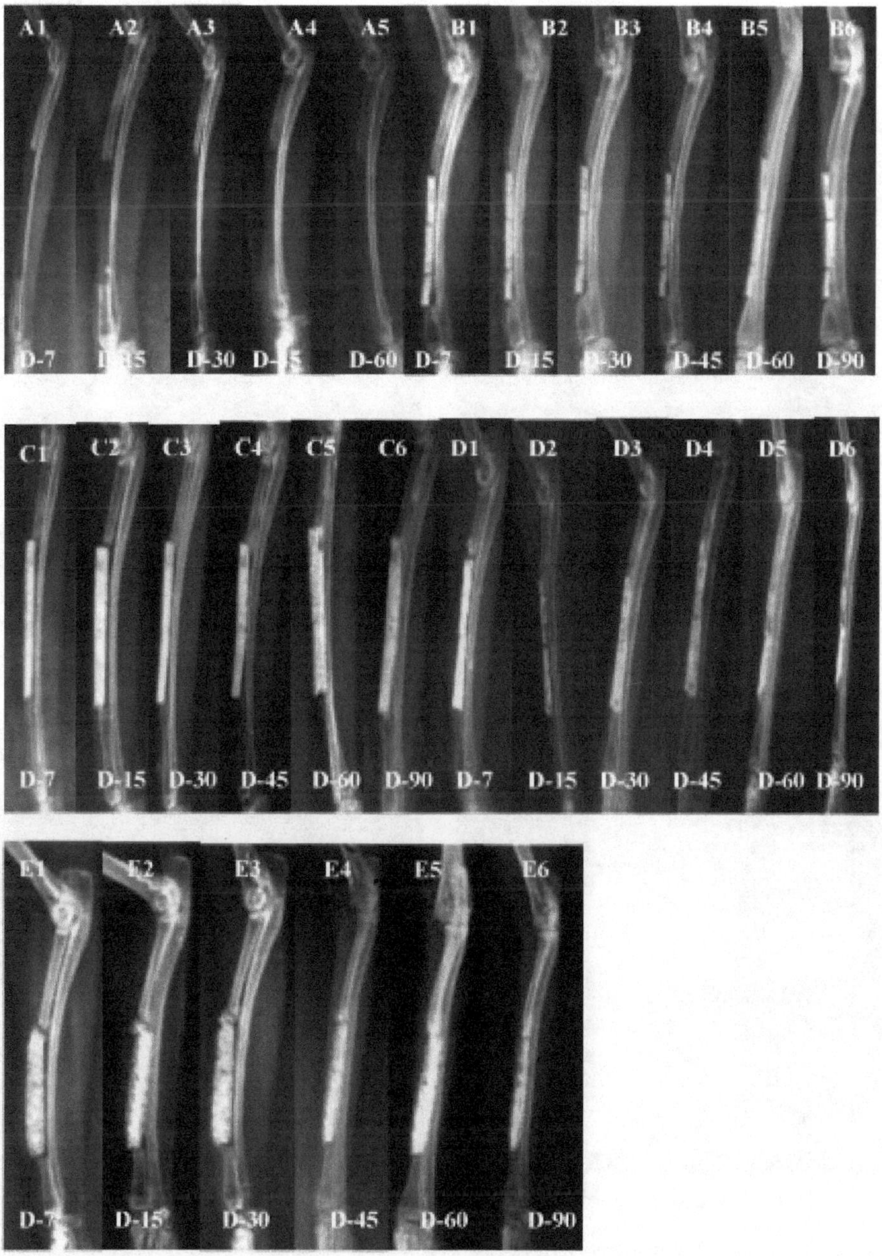

Mediolateral radiographs of groups A, B, C, D and E on Day 7, 15, 30, 45, 60 and 90 days

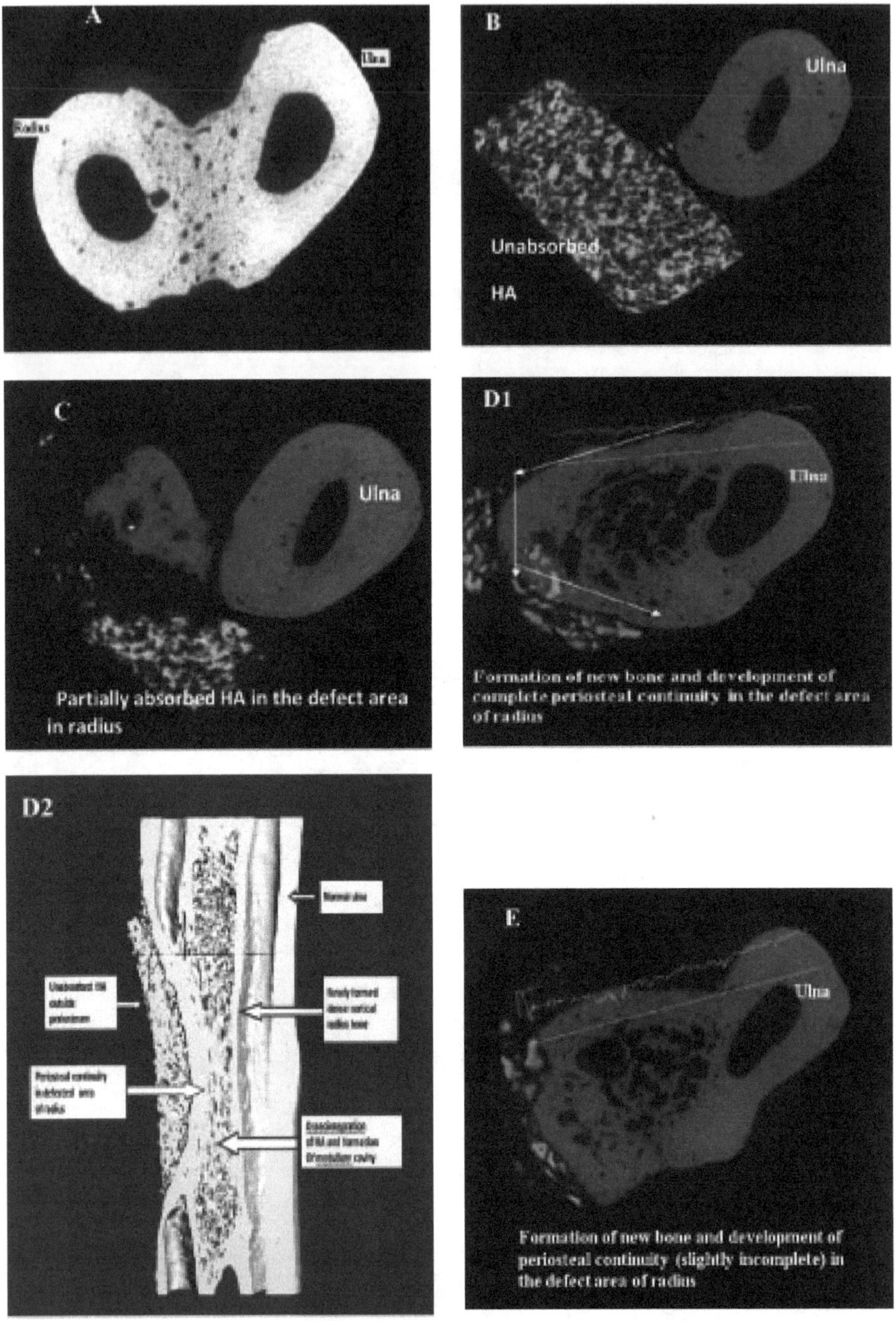

3D transverse bone biopsy slices of groups A, B, C, D and E on day 90

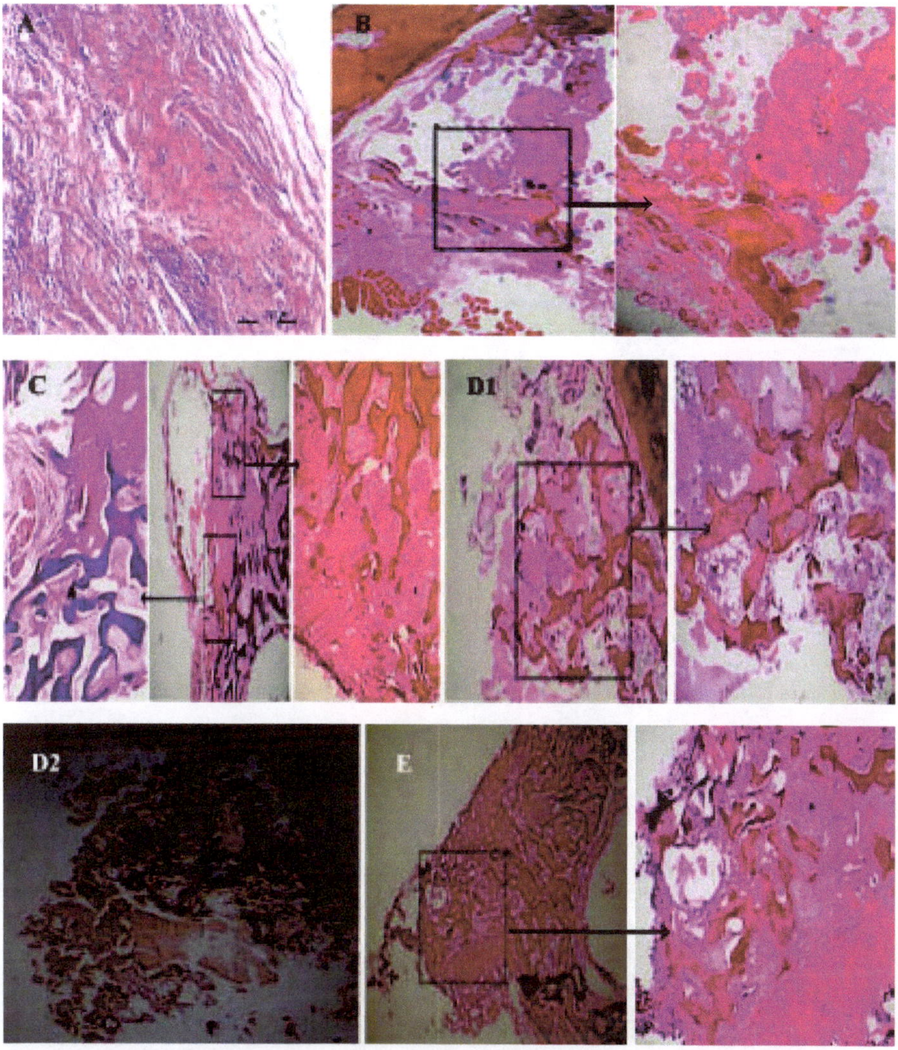

Histopathological section at bone defect site of different groups on day 90

8

Effect of Medical Grade Chitosan Powder with Mesenchymal Stem Cell for Full Thickness Skin Wound Healing in Rat Model

Disruption of the cellular or anatomical continuity of the normal organ structure is known as wound. Healing involves migration, infiltration, proliferation and differentiation of several cell types like keratinocytes, fibroblasts, endothelial cells, macrophages, and platelets which are culminate as an inflammatory response, new tissue formation and wound closure. Healing of the wound starts from the moment of the injury and can continue for varying periods of time depending on the extent of wound. The process of wound healing involves coagulation, inflammation, formation of granulation tissue, matrix formation, remodeling of connective tissue, collagenization and acquisition of wound strength.

Chitosan is a -1, 4-linked polymer of glucosamine (2-amino-2-deoxy—D-glucose) and lesser amounts of N-acetylglucosamine. It is a derivative of chitin (poly-Nacetylglucosamine) which is the second most abundant biopolymer after cellulose. Chitosan is first discovered in 1811 by Henri Braconnota, a French chemist and pharmacist. Later in the century, chitin is found in crustaceans (such as crabs, lobsters, shellfish and shrimp). Chitosan is a biodegradable polymer and it accelerates wound healing. It has been reported that chitosan permits regeneration of tissue elements in skin wounds and has positive application effects on wound healing.

The term mesenchymal stem cell (MSCs) applies to adult fibroblast- like cells that differentiate along multiple mesenchymal pathways when exposed to proper stimuli. Mesenchymal stem cells have demonstrated therapeutic characteristics in wounds and ischemic situations. The therapeutic characteristics of these cells are activated upon their entering wounds or other damaged tissues. Currently there are two basic delivery methods: systemic infusion of the cells into vascular circulation and direct application of therapeutic cells to the wound sites. Upon entering into wounds, therapeutic cells interact with other wound cells through paracrine mechanisms that are not yet well understood. The source of donor tissue can be xenogenic, allogenic, or autogenic. Ideally, both structural and functional tissue replacement will occur with minimal complications. With this background, in this chapter, the potential effect of cultured xenogenic rabbit bone marrow derived mesenchymal stem cells (rBMSC) seeded in medical grade Chitosan powder on full thickness skin wound healing in rat model is described.

The study is conducted in 36 wistar rats in four equal groups to evaluate the wound healing potentiality of medical grade Chitosan powder, mesenchymal stem cells therapy with and without Chitosan for the healing of full thickness skin wounds.

One 2 X 2 cm^2 full thickness skin wound is created on dorsal region of thorax of adult wistar rats of either sex. Topical application of Dermafin gauze over the wound area acts as control (gr I). Full thickness skin wound is treated with Chitosan powder (gr II), xenogenic mesenchymal stem cells (gr III) and mesenchymal stem cells along with Chitosan powder (gr IV). The wound healing are evaluated based on clinical, macroscopical, histopathological, gross observations and photographic evaluations.

This study is performed into three phases. In first phase, collection, isolation and culture of bone marrow derived mesenchymal stem cells (BM-rMSC) from adult New Zealand white rabbit are performed. The aspiration technique from long bones is provided a good amount of bone marrow for culturing of adult mesenchymal stem cells. The cell separation technique as per histopaque protocol resulted in isolation of the mononuclear fraction of bone marrow is very easy. The r-MSCs are cultured over DMEM medium in cell culture flask. The method is used for isolation and culture of r-MSC as described in earlier chapter. Using the same protocol of cell culture, r-MSC took time to reach confluences on 12-14 days. Then these cells are subjected to 3 passages for its therapeutic application.

In the second phase, expansion & characterization of bone marrow derived rabbit mesenchymal stem cells (BM-rMSC) and *in vitro* osteogenic differentiation of BM-rMSC is performed. About four million of cells are taken for expansion & characterization of bone marrow derived rabbit mesenchymal stem cells. They are characterized by mesenchymal stem cells specific markers during proliferation by RT-PCR. Briefly, the procedure includes isolation of RNA from rabbit mesenchymal stem cell; C-DNA preparation from isolated r-RNA, PCR from CD-105, CD-44, CD-73, CD-34 and CD-45 and Beta Actin specific (House keepng gene) specific primers, agarose gel electrophoresis (1% agarose).

It is concluded that rabbit adult mesenchymal stem cells are positive for CD-105, CD-73, CD-44, whereas, it is expressed negative for CD-34 and CD-45. To characterize unique differentiating property of rMSC and mineral deposition, osteogenic differentiation is performed in monolayer culture for 3 weeks after adding osteogenic supplementation media. After 3 weeks of culture, the induced cells morphology is changed and is stain positive with Alizarin red S stain for mineral deposition in their newly formed matrix. Control cultures, although becoming over-confluence after 3 weeks, retain their fibroblast like appearance, do not formed cell aggregates and are stain negative for mineral deposition.

In the third phase, wound healing potentiality of medical grade Chitosan powder with or without xenogenic mesenchymal stem cell is evaluated in the excisional full thickness skin wound in rat model. Wounds are photographs on days 0, 3, 7, 14, 21 and 28 post-surgery and evaluated by independent observers to assess the quality of wound healing and cosmetic outcome.

The animals of all the groups remain dull on first postoperative day and assumed a hunched back posture, while resting in their individual cages. Animals of different groups start taking feed and water partially within 24h after surgery. In all the animals feed and water intake become normal by 3rd postoperative day. Significant increase in temperature for first 3 days post surgery is recorded which may be due to foreign body reaction, surgical trauma and stress to the animals following skin wound. Wound heals completely by 28 days leaving a large scar indicates the existence of severe contraction in control group. In Chitosan group (II), it takes about 25-26 days for complete healing with minimum contraction and little scar formation in comparison to control group. The higher rate of wound healing with minimum contraction and minimum scar formation is found in groups III and IV than groups I and II. This may be due to the added effects of bone marrow derived mesenchymal stem cells. In group III and IV, wound heals completely on day 23-24 and day 20-21 respectively. Moderate exudation at the site is observed up to day 3-5 in all the treated as well as control groups. However, animals of group I and group II shows significantly higher values of exudation on days 3 and 6 respectively as compared to groups III and group IV. Although moderate degree of postoperative pain persist up to day 6 in all the groups but pain scores is non-significant among different groups. In all the groups the pain scores reduce gradually and reach to minimum level on day 7. Granulation tissue is first observed in group IV followed by groups III, II and I. Granulation tissue formation is almost same in groups II and III on day 7. Granulation tissue formation is not so significant on day 14 in group I. Granulation tissue is almost fully covered the wound area in groups II, III and IV on day 21. However, excellent granulation tissue formation and completion of wound healing is found in group IV on day 21. No scar formation is noticed in group IV on day 21. Degree of peripheral swelling is less in group IV in comparison to control group, because both Chitosan powder and stem cell have anti-inflammatory action. Wound contraction study provides a definite clue for the effectiveness of the treatment which reveals a gradual decrease in the size of the wounds. Progressive increase in percent of wound contraction is recorded in all the groups, however, in group IV, wound contraction is faster.

Histopathological examinations are conducted on the biopsy samples collected on 7th, 14th, and 28th day post surgery. Biopsy samples are examined with routine H&E staining and special staining for collagen with Masson Trichome staining. In terms of surface epithelium presence and thickness, the wounds with group IV shows early epithelization with an early proliferation of fibroblast and angioblast cells to fill the defect. This group also shows an early resemblance to the normal skin than other groups. On day 7, inflammatory reaction is more pronounced in group I than groups II, III and IV may be due to anti-inflammatory and anti-bacterial effects of Chitosan and mesenchymal stem cells. On day 14, this inflammatory reaction further reduce in the treatment groups II, III and IV; whereas in group I, mild neutrophil infiltration still is observed. Scanty granulation tissue and collagen fibers are observed in all the groups on the 7th day post wounding. There is a rapid reduction in the granulation tissue which is found from day 14 to 21 in groups III and IV with a simultaneous increase in the collagen secretion. Thin, less dense and an unorganized collagen fibre arrangement is noticed in group I on day 28 whereas, it is more dense, thick and organized in treatment groups viz, groups, II and III. In group IV, this picture of dense, uniformly arranged collagen fibre is found perfect and best on day 28. Epithelisation is more uniformed and complete in groups II, III and IV than group I on day 28.

In conclusion, medical grade Chitosan powder has better healing potentiality than standard dressing materials for repair of full thickness skin wound. Stem cells treated group shows better healing potentiality than Chitosan powder alone but mesenchymal stem cells therapy adjunct with Chitosan powder prove best among all the groups. Xenogenic stem cells prove as immune privileged as evidenced by clinical and histopathological observations.

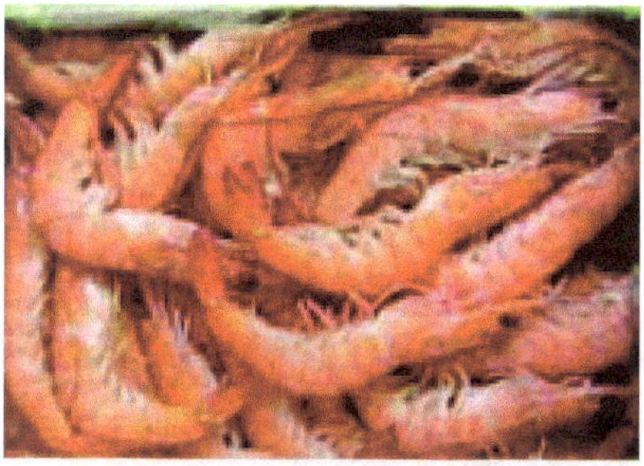 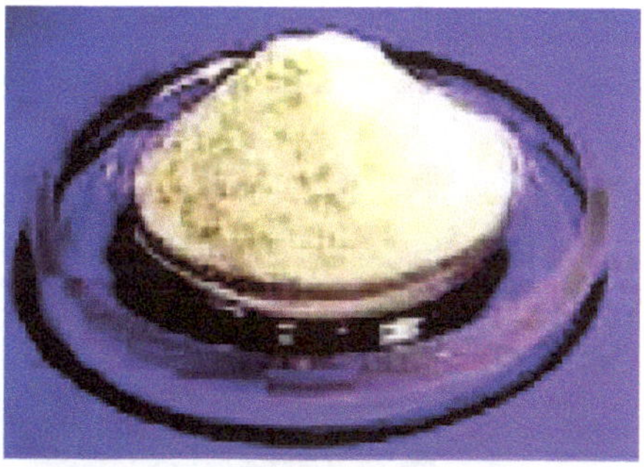

Natural biomaterial-chitosan powder (medical grade)

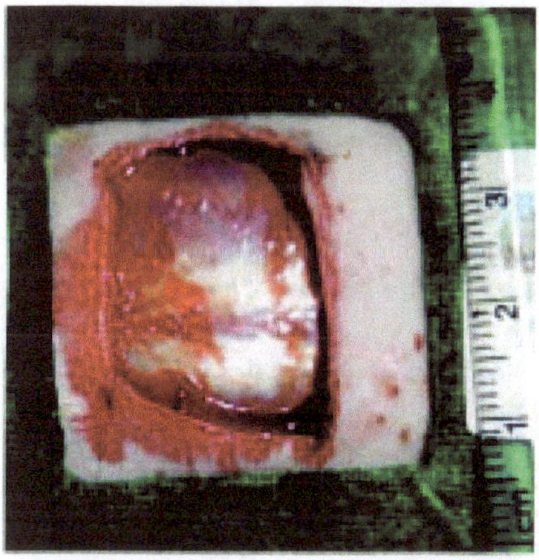

Creation of skin wound ($2x2cm^2$)

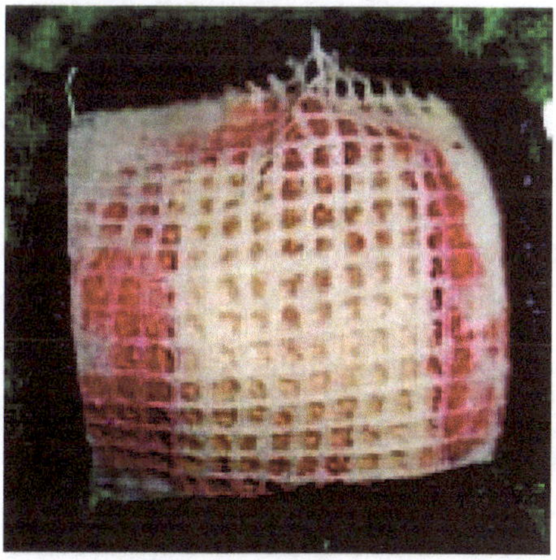

Paraffin gauze dressing

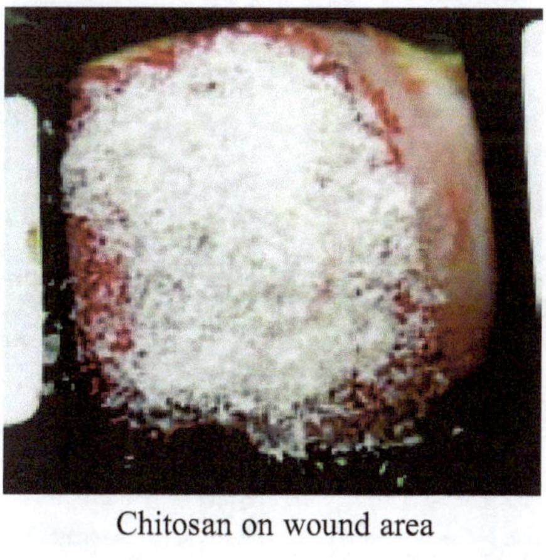

Chitosan on wound area

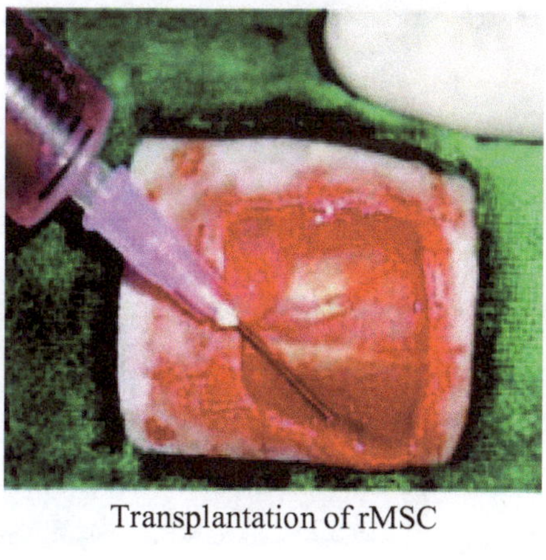

Transplantation of rMSC

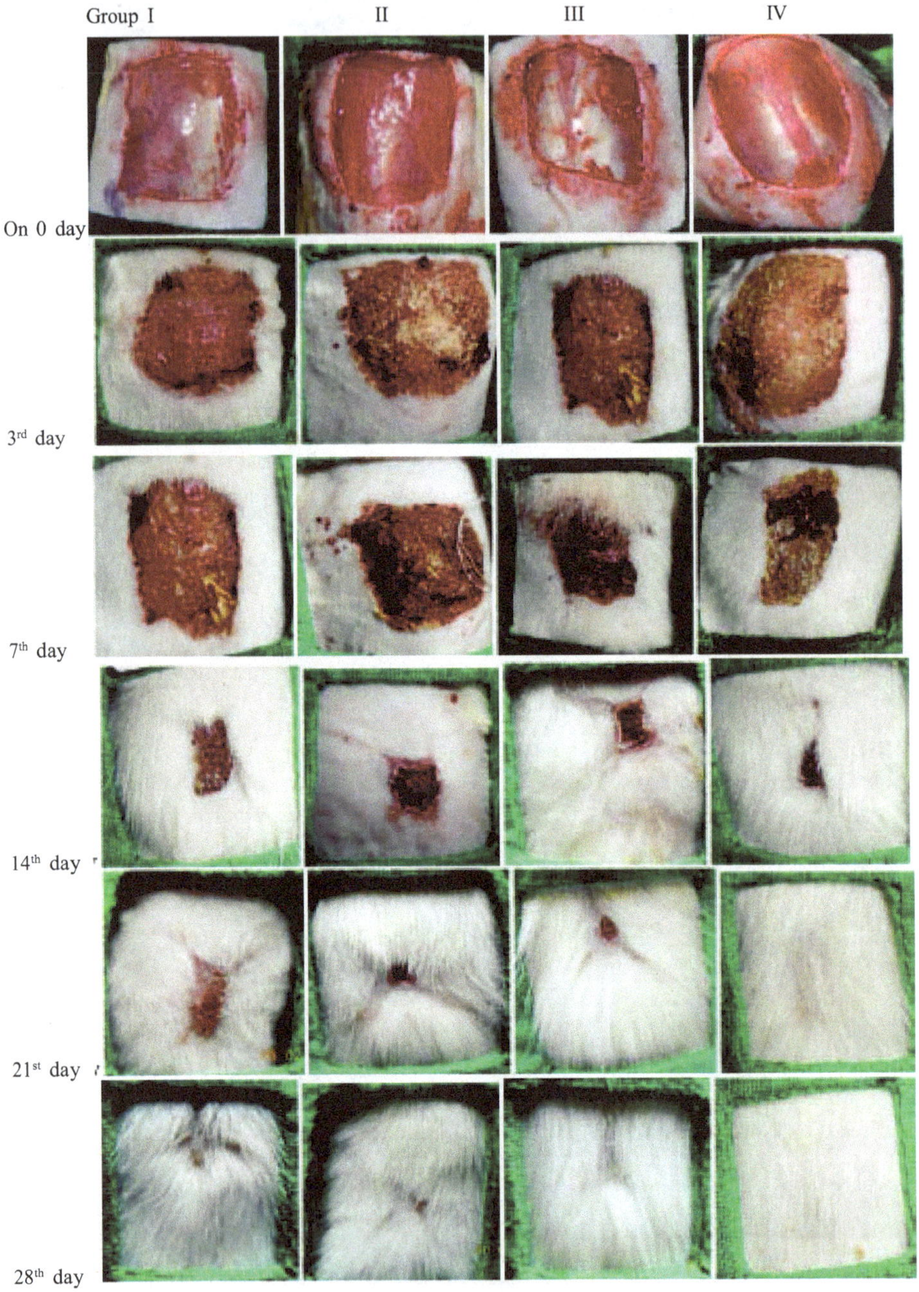

Colour digital image processing

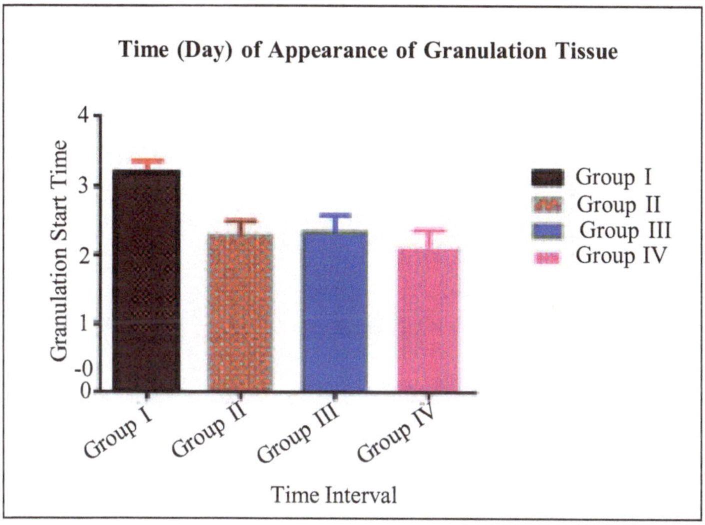

Mean + S.E values of time (day) of appearance of granulation tissue

Histopathology

Gr-I Gr-II Gr-III Gr-IV

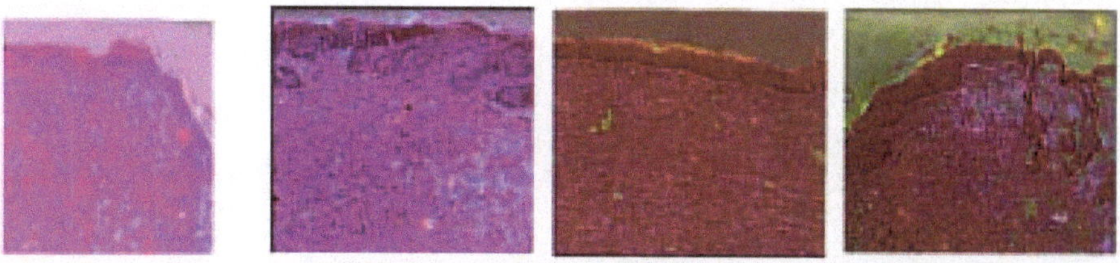

H&E Staining

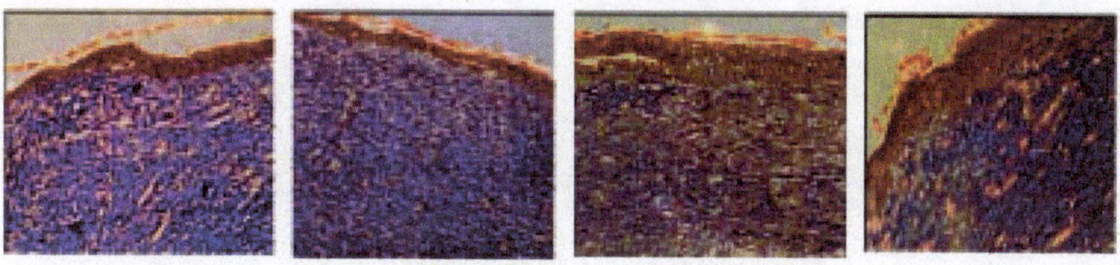

Masson Trichrome Staining

9

Evaluation of Mesenchymal Stem Cell Seeded Decellularized Porcine Intestine and Decellularized Cornea for the Repair of Corneal Defect in Rabbit Model

The cornea is the anterior transparent part of the fibrous tunic of the globe which has both mechanical and optical function. It functions to support the intraocular contents and transmit and refract light. Histologically, the cornea is composed of an outer stratified squamous corneal epithelium and its basement membrane, an underlying collagenous stroma, a thin acellular membrane, and an inner monolayer of cells, the corneal endothelium. In dogs, the central cornea is thinner than the peripheral cornea, whereas regional differences in thickness may not exist in cats. The active pumping mechanism of corneal endothelium and the barrier function of anterior epithelium keep the cornea in a state of relative dehydration. Compromise of either of these mechanisms will allow corneal edema to develop, with a concomitant increase in corneal thickness. Corneal ulceration is one of the most common ophthalmic disorders in veterinary medicine. Corneal ulcers are classified based on depth and ease of healing. There are several phases during the corneal epithelial wound healing process, including a lag phase where cells alter their metabolic status; a migration phase to cover the bare surface; a proliferation phase and a differentiation phase, where cells stratify and re-establish multiple layers of distinct cells. Methods of surgical treatment for canine corneal ulcers include temporary tarsorrhaphy, third eyelid flap, conjunctival pedicle graft, tissue adhesive, corneo-scleral graft and transplantation of natural or synthetic material.

Scaffolds derived from processed tissues offer viable alternatives to synthetic polymers as biological scaffolds for regenerative medicine. Tissue-derived scaffolds provides an extracellular matrix as the starting material for wound healing and the functional reconstruction of tissues, offering a potentially valuable approach for the replacement of damaged or missing tissues. Additionally, acellular tissue may provide a natural microenvironment for host-cell migration and the induction of stem cell differentiation to contribute for tissue regeneration.

Small intestinal submucosa (SIS) is derived from the sub-mucosal layer of the jejunum and consists of the stratum compactum layer of the tunica mucosa, the tunica muscularis mucosa, and the tunica submucosa. This biomaterial is primarily an acellular extracellular matrix composed of collagen, proteoglycans, glycoproteins, and glycosaminoglycans. It also contains natural growth factors including basic fibroblast growth factor and transforming growth factor beta. SIS has several interesting physical and biological properties: it has good tensile properties, non-immunogenic, resistant to infection and when used as a xenograft material it promotes wound healing by providing a scaffold for tissue in growth. After implantation, the collagen matrix is degraded and is replaced by an autologous tissue that closely resembles the native structure.

The cornea itself has a unique ECM organization which provides significant mechanical properties in addition to innate biological cues which help to direct and organize cell function, including cell differentiation, proliferation and migration. Decellularization protocols include several steps to promote the lyses of the cell membrane, separate the cellular components from the ECM, solubilize the cytoplasmic and nuclear-cellular components, and remove the cellular debris from the tissue. The decellularization treatments largely preserve the native structure of the stromal collagen, with orthogonally arranged collagen fibrils, a textured appearance of Bowman's layer and the fiber-like structure of Descemet's membrane.

The term mesenchymal stem cell (MSCs) applies to adult fibroblast- like cells that differentiate along multiple mesenchymal pathways when exposed to proper stimuli. Mesenchymal stem cells have demonstrated therapeutic characteristics in wounds and ischemic situations. The therapeutic characteristics of these cells are activated upon their entering wounds or other damaged tissues. These cells are expanded in culture, attached to a support matrix, and then re-implanted into the host after expansion. Cells can also be use for therapy through injection, either with carriers such as hydrogels or alone.

Tissue engineering is the use of combination of cells, engineering and suitable biochemical and physio-chemical factors to improve or replace biological functions. Tissue engineering has progressed rapidly in recent years and has now emerged as a potential alternative to tissue or organ transplantation. Tissue engineering of adult mesenchymal stem cells seeded with acellular biomaterials have been used successfully in full thickness skin wound repair in different species of animals.

In this chapter, healing potentiality of mesenchymal stem cells seeded decellularized porcine small intestinal submucosa and cornea in lamellar keratectomy wound in rabbit model is described.

Freshly collected porcine small intestine and eyes from the local abattoir is cleaned thoroughly by washing in sterile physiological normal saline. Cornea is separated and placed in sterile PBS. The serosa and muscular layer of small intestine is removed by gentle scrapping. The prepared scaffolds are cut into 1x1 cm^2 pieces and keep in sterile PBS containing antibiotics for 2 h at room temperature. Decellularization of porcine cornea and small intestine are done by treating it with 1% SDS in an orbital shaker for 12 h. These decellularized scaffolds are thoroughly washed in PBS solution and stored at -20°C in PBS containing antibiotics. These tissues are subjected to histological and scanning electron microscopic (SEM) examination to check their acellularity.

Allogenic bone marrow derived rabbit mesenchymal stem cells (rBM-MSCs) are collected, cultured and expanded as described in previous chapter. The third passage cells are used for seeding on decellularized SIS and cornea. For preparation of bioengineered scaffold, cells are cultured on the tissue scaffolds keep in 6 well plate containing DMEM for 14 days. Attachment of mesenchymal stem cells on the scaffold is confirmed by histopathology and scanning electron microscopy. The bioengineered scaffolds are compared with the decellularized porcine small intestinal submucosa and decellularized porcine cornea alone.

The study is conducted in thirty clinically healthy adult New Zealand white rabbits of either sex divided equally in six groups. In all groups, a 5 mm diameter partial thickness corneal defect is made for assessing the healing potential of tissue engineered scaffolds.

Treatment is given to different groups of animals as follows:

Groups	Treatment
A	No treatment for corneal defect (control)
B	Corneal defect is repaired with decellularized porcine cornea
C	Corneal defect is repaired with r-MSC seeded decellularized porcine cornea
D	Corneal defect is repaired with decellularized small intestinal submucosa (SIS)
E	Corneal defect is repaired with r-MSC seeded small intestinal submucosa (SIS)

Animals are anaesthetized with Xylazine @ 5mg/kg and Ketamine @ 50 mg/kg body weight given intramuscularly. The animals are restrained in lateral recumbency. The right eye is selected in all cases for surgical procedure. The eyelashes are clipped and periorbital area is cleaned with Povidone iodine solution. Procedures are done under strict aseptic conditions. After trephining the cornea with a corneal trephine of 5 mm diameter, a partial thickness defect is created on the peripheral cornea in all the groups. The defect in different groups is immediately repaired with appropriate sized scaffolds as per Table above. In control group of animals (A) the defect is left untreated. In animals of treatment groups, scaffolds are implanted on to the cornea by synthetic absorbable suture material. In all groups tarsorrhaphy is performed by using nylon. Systemic and local broad-spectrum antibiotic and anti-inflammatory drugs are given for 5 days postoperatively. Tarsorrhaphy suture is removed on 15th postoperative day.

The efficacy of the bio-engineered scaffolds for the reconstruction of corneal defects is evaluated based on the following parameters. The animals are observed for corneal healing by serial subjective evaluation of cornea on 15, 30, 45 and 60 days postoperatively. After euthanizing the animals on 15, 30, 45, and 60 days the healing is evaluated by histopathological examination.

Corneal healing and vision: The healing status and the gross appearance of corneal defects are examined by an independent observer after removal of tarsorrhaphy sutures, based on the following parameters and the examination is repeated on 30, 45 and 60thday: I) Conjunctival injection and chemosis, II) Oedema of peripheral cornea and iritis characterized by miosis and iridial hyperemia, III) Transparency of cornea, IV) Fluorescein and Rose Bengal staining of cornea, V) Schirmer tears testing, VI) Pupillary and menace reflexes, VII) Blink reflex and VIII) Corneal neovascularization.

Computerized planimetry: Colour photographs are taken and analyze subjectively for healing status on day 15, 30, 45 and 60th post operatively by an independent observer.

For histopathological studies, the treated cornea is collected from the animals sacrificed on days 15, 30, 45 and 60 days postoperatively. The cornea is washed thoroughly in normal saline and fixed in 10% buffered formalin for 48–72 hours and is processed in routine manner for H & E staining as per the standard procedure. For Immunological studies, estimation of protein contents, indirect ELISA for antibody detection in rabbit serum at different post-implantation period and lymphocyte stimulation test is carried out.

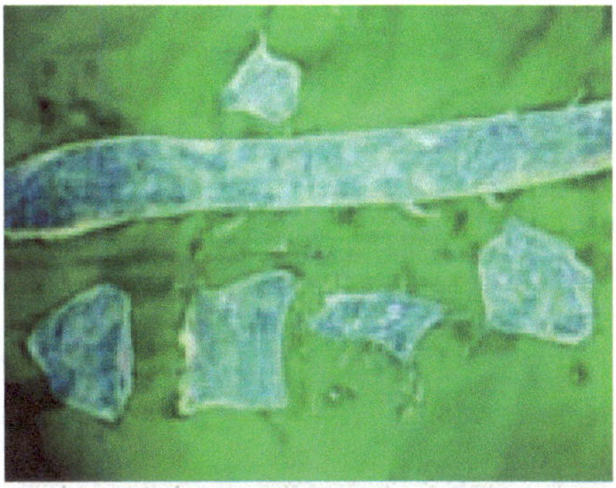

Native porcine small intestinal submucosa

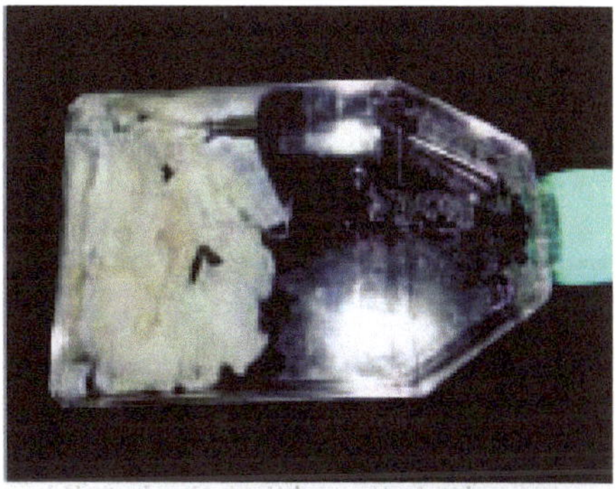

Decellularized small intestinal submucosa

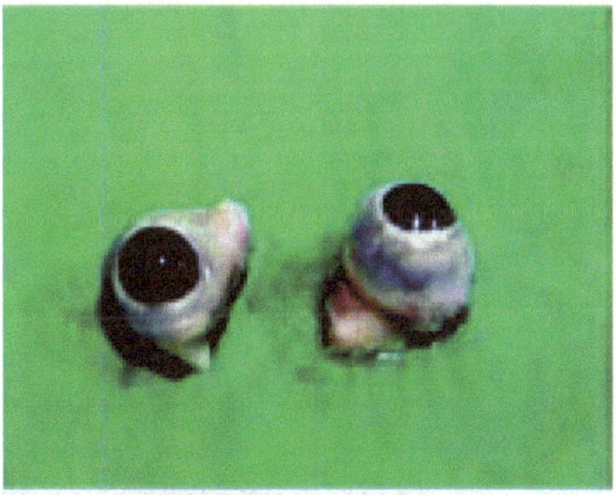

Enucleated porcine eye ball

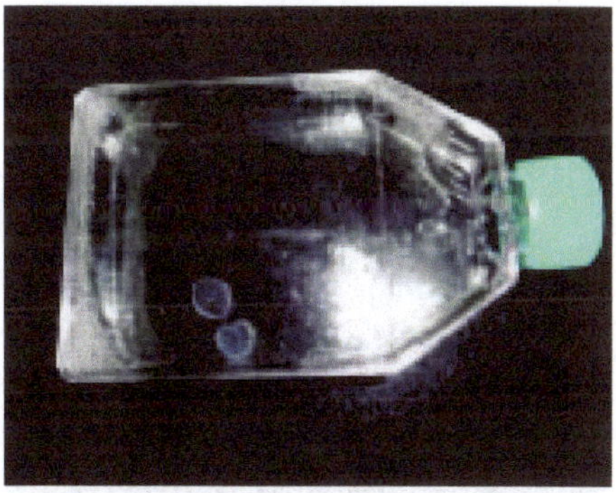

Decellularized porcine cornea

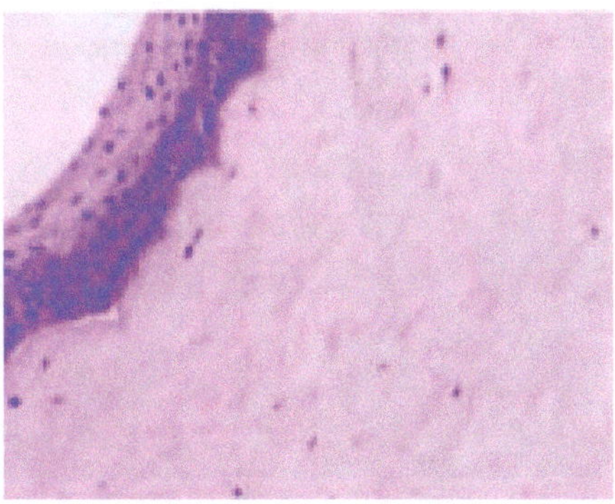

Histology of native porcine cornea

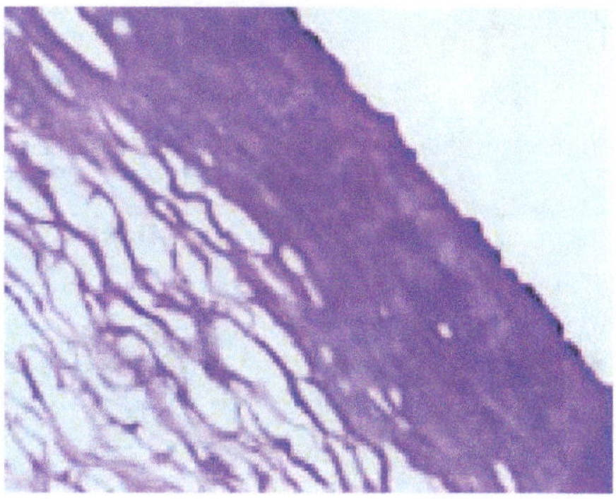

Histology of decellularized porcine cornea

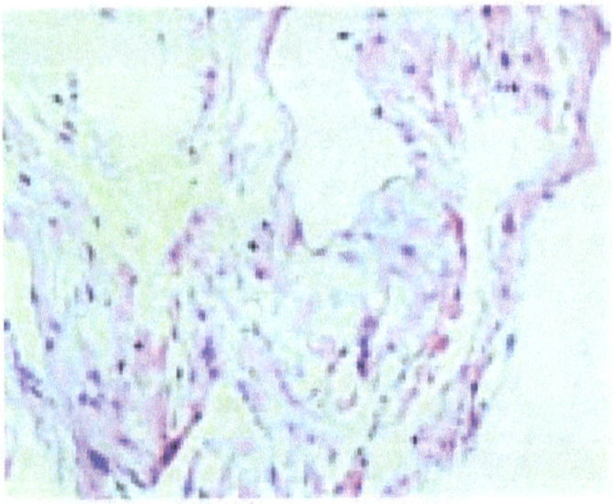

Histology of native porcine SIS

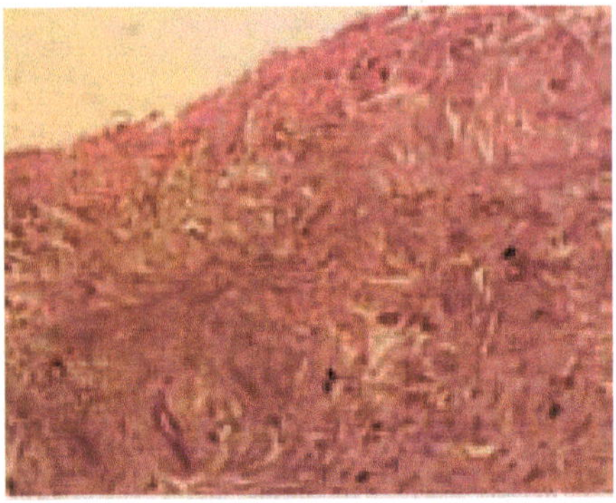

Histology of decellularized porcine SIS

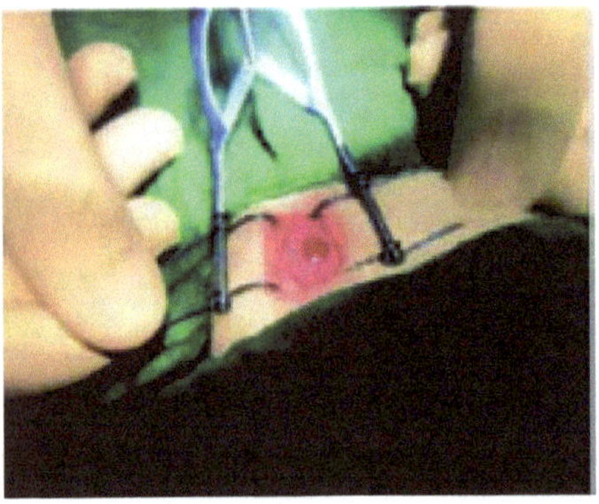

Eye speculum in position

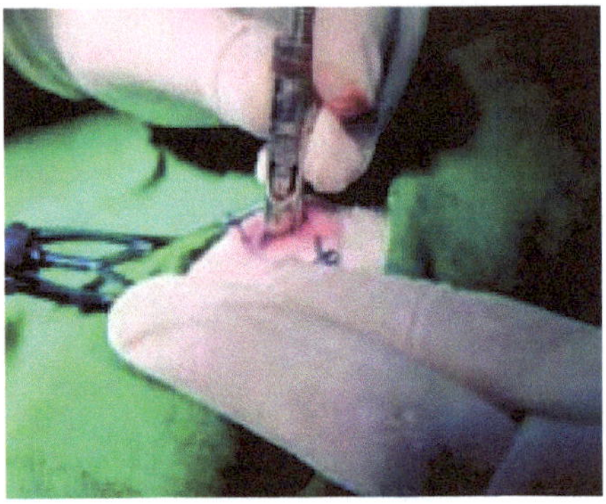

Trephining of cornea

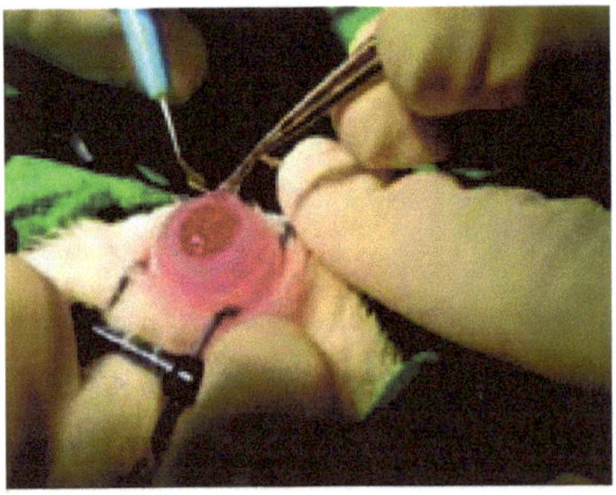

Lamellar keratectomy

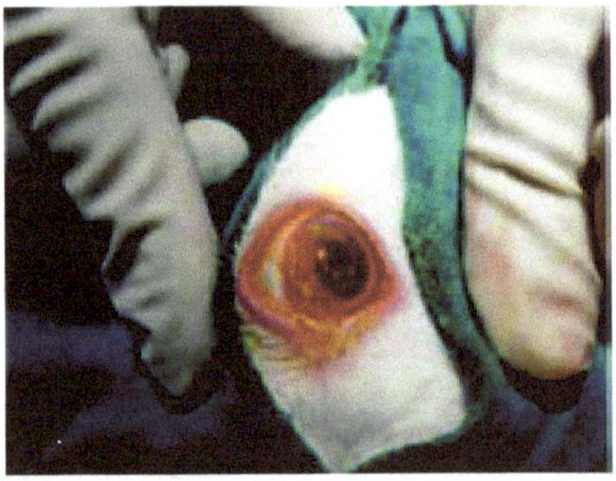

Staining with fluorescein stain

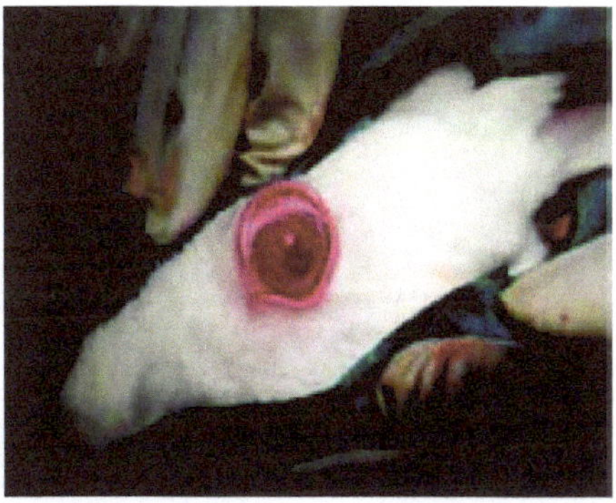

Staining with Rose Bengal stain

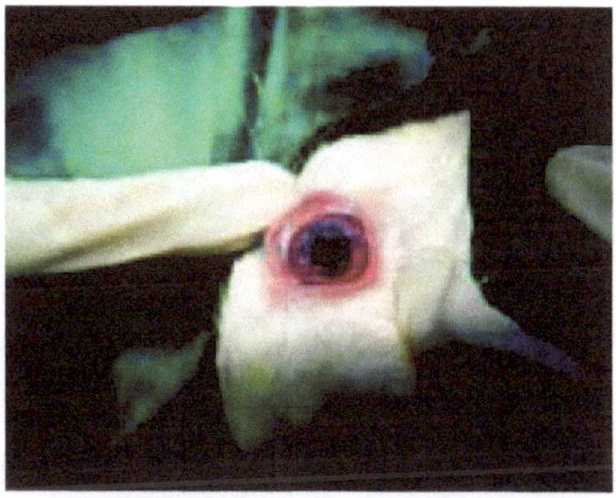

Staining with lissamine green stain

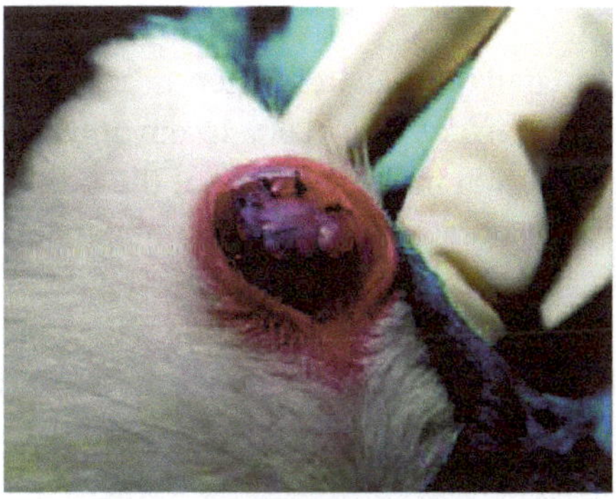

Defect repaired with decellularized cornea

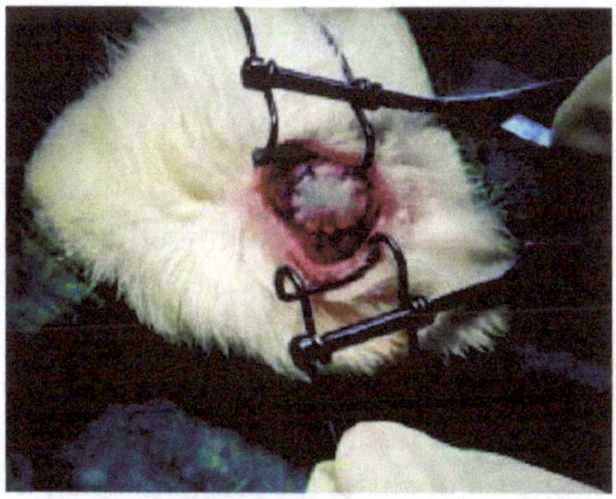

Defect repaired with decellularized SIS

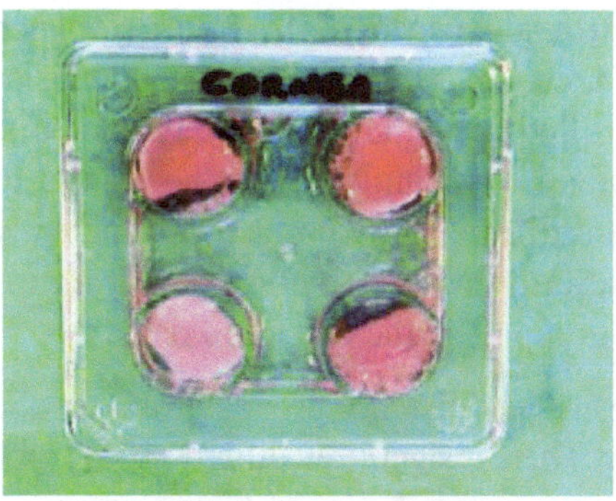

r-MSC seeded scaffolds

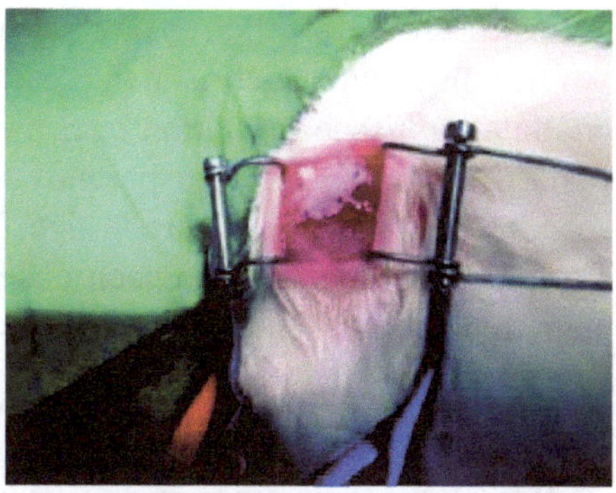

Defect repaired with r-MSC seeded decellularized SIS

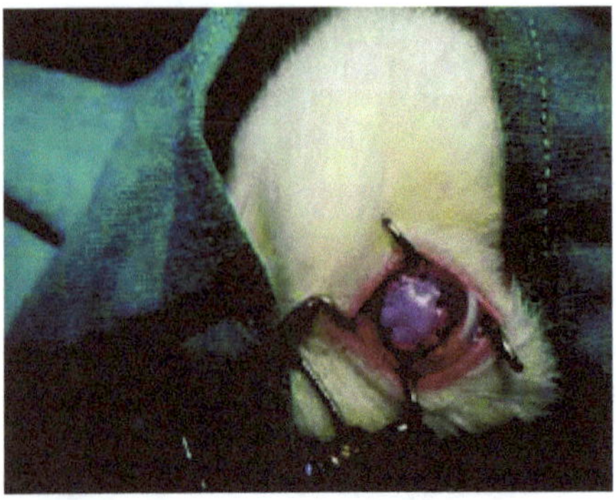

Defect repaired with r-MSC seeded decellularized cornea

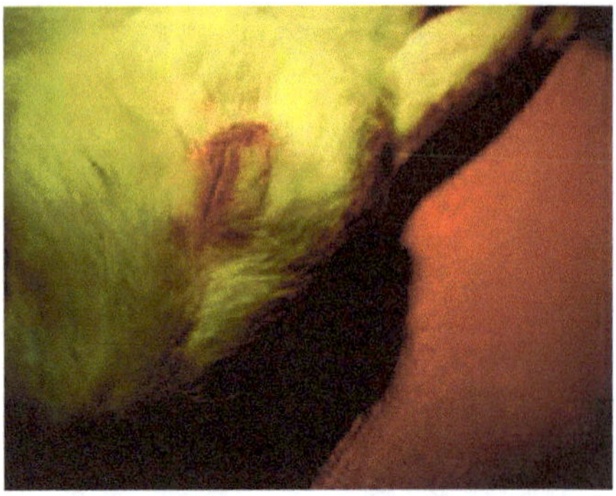

After tarsorrhaphy

Result

The healing status of corneal wound is evaluated immediately after the removal of tarsorrhaphy sutures on day 15th postoperative day and every 15 day interval thereafter. There is no sign of infection or stromal melting in any of the group. Maximum conjunctival injection and chemosis is scored by day 15, immediately after the removal of tarsorrhaphy sutures in all the groups. Thereafter a gradual decrease is observed in different groups. Significant conjunctival injection and chemosis is observed by day 15 in group B and group D. Among the grafted groups conjunctival injection and chemosis is comparatively lower in group C. Immediately after the removal of tarsorrhaphy sutures, maximum corneal edema and iridial hyperemia is recorded in all groups. Thereafter no significant difference is recorded in any of the groups on the following observation days. The xenograft is opalescent and swollen by day 15. Superficial layers of the grafts are sloughed off forming whitish debris in the grafted area. On 30th day there is evidence of granulation tissue formation over the grafted area and by 45th day cornea is started regaining the transparency. Extend of granulation tissue is less in group C and group E. There is significant difference in corneal transparency between all the groups on each observation interval. Among grafted groups maximum corneal clarity is recorded in group C by the end of 60 days.

There is no significant difference observed between any groups at any of the observation intervals for fluorescein staining. There is significant difference in degree of Rose Bengal staining on day 30 between group A, group C and group D. On all observation days, degree of dye retention is lesser in group C than in other groups. In Schirmer tear test, initially there is an increased tear production in all the experimental groups which gradually decrease during subsequent intervals. However, in none of the groups it reaches the normal value. Significant difference in pupillary light reflex is observed in all the grafted groups on day 15 and day 30. Afterwards, pupillary reflex is recorded normal in all the groups. In menace reflex, significant difference is observed only on 15th day between the control group and all the grafted groups. In all the treatment groups the scaffold on the cornea imposes a hindrance for the normal vision. However, when the grafted material is resorbed the menace reflex becomes normal. In blink reflex, on day 15, varying amount of grafted material is still present over the cornea in different treatment groups and there is significant difference in blink reflex between control group and all the grafted groups. Afterwards blink reflex gradually become normal in all the treatment groups.

Corneal neovascularization is evident in all the grafted group of animals and it is significantly higher on all the observation intervals when compare to the control group where no graft is placed. Degree of neovascularization is highest by day 30. Thereafter number of blood vessels over the cornea starts decreasing. By day 60 only two to three blood vessels are there and those blood vessels are extended up to the centre of the cornea. Among the grafted groups neovascularization is comparatively less in group C.

The cell mediated immune response towards xenogenic scaffolds in all the experimental animals is assessing by colorimetric assay. The stimulation of rabbit lymphocytes with phytohaemaglutinin is considered as positive control, whereas unstimulated cell culture is taken as negative control. Blood is collected on day 0, 45 and 60 for separating lymphocytes. The lymphocyte culture is performed to grow cells *in-vitro.* These lymphocytes are stimulated with native porcine cornea antigen and PHA. On day 45 group B shows significantly higher stimulation index against native porcine cornea antigen. The stimulation index is less in group C and group E where the scaffolds are seeded with rabbit mesenchymal stem cells. Thereafter a decrease in stimulation index is observed.

The humoral immune response elicited by the implanted xenogenic scaffolds in different grafted groups is determined by indirect ELISA. Native porcine cornea is used as coating antigen. The serum samples collected on day 0, 15, 30, 45 and 60 post implantation are evaluated for the levels of antibody generated towards the implanted scaffolds. The levels of antibodies present in serum prior to implantation are taken as basal values. By day 15 the immune response is significantly higher in group B and group D. In all the grafted groups there is increased in antibody titer by day 30 and day 45 post implantation and it is significantly higher in group D when compare to group A and C. When compare to non-seeded groups, the immune response is less in group C and group E, where the scaffolds are seeded with mesenchymal stem cells. Thereafter no significant difference is observed in immune response in any of the group.

The animals are euthanized on day 15, 30, 45 and 60 postoperatively and cornea is collected in 10% formalin. The samples are then processed for hematoxylin and eosin staining. In group A, by 15th day signs of epithelial regeneration is observed. The newly formed collagen fibers in stroma are loosely arranged. The nuclei of the anterior epithelium are hyperchromatic and there is neovascularization with presence of lymphocytes in the stroma. By 30th day, stromal collagen fibers become more compact with much more lymphocytes, higher neovascularization and severe inflammatory reaction. By 45th day the extent of neovascularization is less and the stromal tissue seems to be immature when compare with normal tissue. By 60th day the stromal tissue appear loose with neovascularization.

In group B, by 15th day complete regeneration of the lining epithelium with normal arrangement of cells is observed. Subepithelial stromal tissue reveals focal infiltration of lymphocytes, mild to moderate neovascularization and loosely arrange collagen fibers with moderate fibroblastic activity. By 30th day, the anterior epithelium shows complete regeneration with mild increase in thickness. Subepithelial stromal tissue shows severe fibroblastic activity and severe lymphocyte reaction. Neovascular tissue is congested with focal hemorrhages. By 45th day the anterior epithelium appears to be normal with little increase in thickness. Subepithelial stromal tissue shows presence of loosely arranged collagen fibers with occasional presence of lymphocytes, mild fibroblastic activity and presence of few newly formed blood capillaries. By 60th day, anterior epithelium appears normal with normal thickness and regular arrangement of cells. Subepithelial stromal tissue shows loose to dense connective tissue fibers with mild neovascularization and lymphocyte and fibroblastic reaction.

In group C, by day 15 the anterior epithelium reveals complete regeneration and is moderately thickened with regularly arranged cells. Subepithelial stromal tissue shows loosely arranged collagen fibers with moderate lymphocyte infiltration and fibroblastic activity. By day 30, the anterior epithelium appears normal with regular arrangement of cells. Subepithelial stromal tissue appears moderately dense with mild neovascularization and mild lymphocyte and fibroblastic activity. By day 45, anterior epithelium shows normal appearance with normal thickness. Subepithelial stromal tissue appears moderately dense with mild neovascularization and mild lymphocyte and fibroblastic activity. By day 60, the appearance of cornea is similar to that of normal cornea with moderately dense stromal collagen fibers.

In group D, by day 15, the grafted area shows severe neovascularization with incomplete epithelialisation and loose scarce stromal tissue. By day 30, the thickness of epithelium is variable with irregularly arranged cells. The subepithelial stromal tissue shows comparatively dense arrangement of collagen fibers with presence of fibroblasts, mononuclear cells and congested blood vessels. By day 45, the anterior epithelium appears normal with normal arrangement of cells. The corneal stroma shows the presence of less dense collagen fibers with congested blood vessels, focal hemorrhage, lymphocyte infiltration and mild fibroblastic activity. By day 60, the anterior epithelium appears normal with regular cell arrangement but at places shows degeneration with disruption of cells and breach in continuity.

In group E, by day 15, the anterior epithelium shows regeneration with normal arrangement of cells at most places and irregularly arranged cells at other places. Subepithelial stromal tissue shows neovascularization, loose collagen fibers, mild to moderate fibroblastic activity and infiltration of lymphocytes. By day 30, anterior lining epithelium shows apparently normal arrangement of cells with some sort of irregularities at places. Subepithelial stroma reveals loosely arranged collagen fibers with mild to moderate lymphocyte reaction, mild proliferation of fibroblasts and neovascularization. By day 45, the anterior lining epithelium appears normal with regular cell arrangement. Subepithelial stromal tissue reveals presence of normal and dense collagen fibers with occasional presence of lymphocytes and mild fibroblast proliferation. By day 60, anterior epithelium appears normal with regularly arranged cells. Subepithelial stromal tissue shows apparently normal arrangement of collagen fibers with mild lymphocytic reaction and moderate fibroblastic activity.

According to histopathological findings, among the grafted groups, group C is observed to have better healing. Among all the treatment groups, scoring of corneal neovascularization, fibroblast proliferation, arrangement of corneal epithelial cells, leukocyte infiltration and corneal epithelial thickening reveals corneal healing is best in group C, where corneal defect is repaired with rMSC seeded decellularization porcine cornea. In all the treatment groups, there is no evidence of any sign of rejection in any of the grafted group.

In conclusion, decellularized porcine cornea is found to have better healing potential than decellularized porcine small intestinal submucosa for the repair of corneal defect in rabbits and seeding of allogenic mesenchymal stem cells (r-MSCs) on decellularized porcine cornea enhance its healing potential for the repair of corneal defect in rabbits and allogenic MSCs prove as immune privileged.

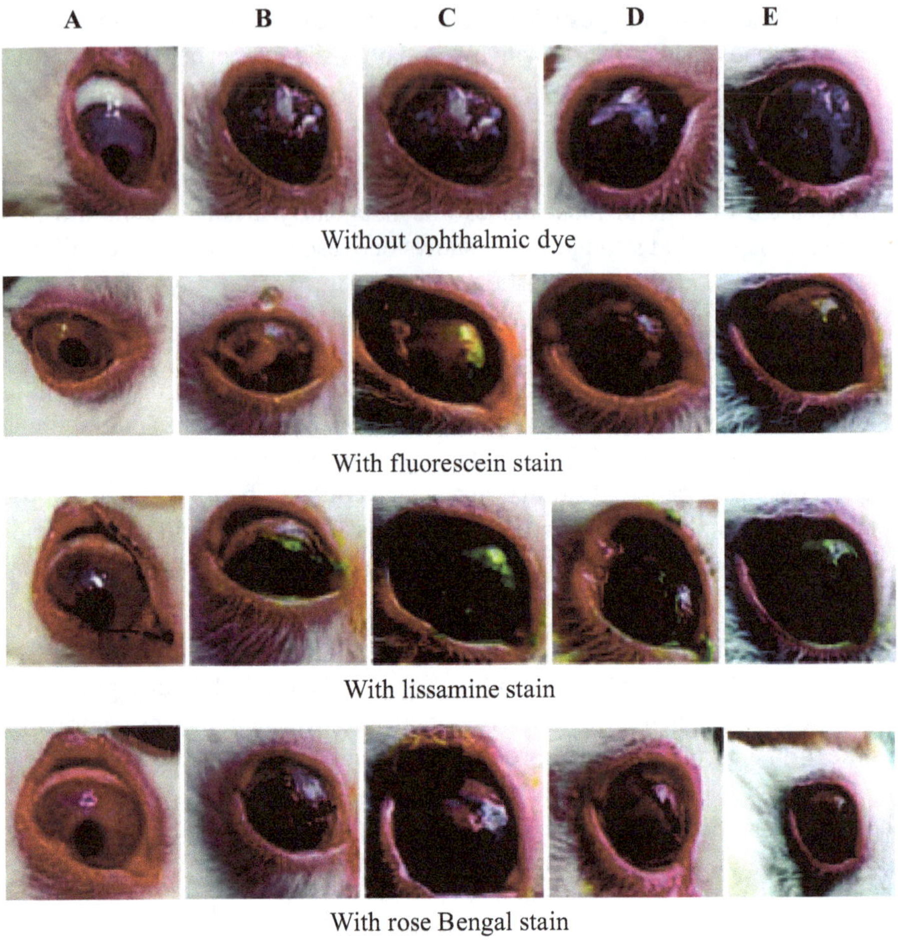

Colour photographs of treated groups on day 15 post implantation

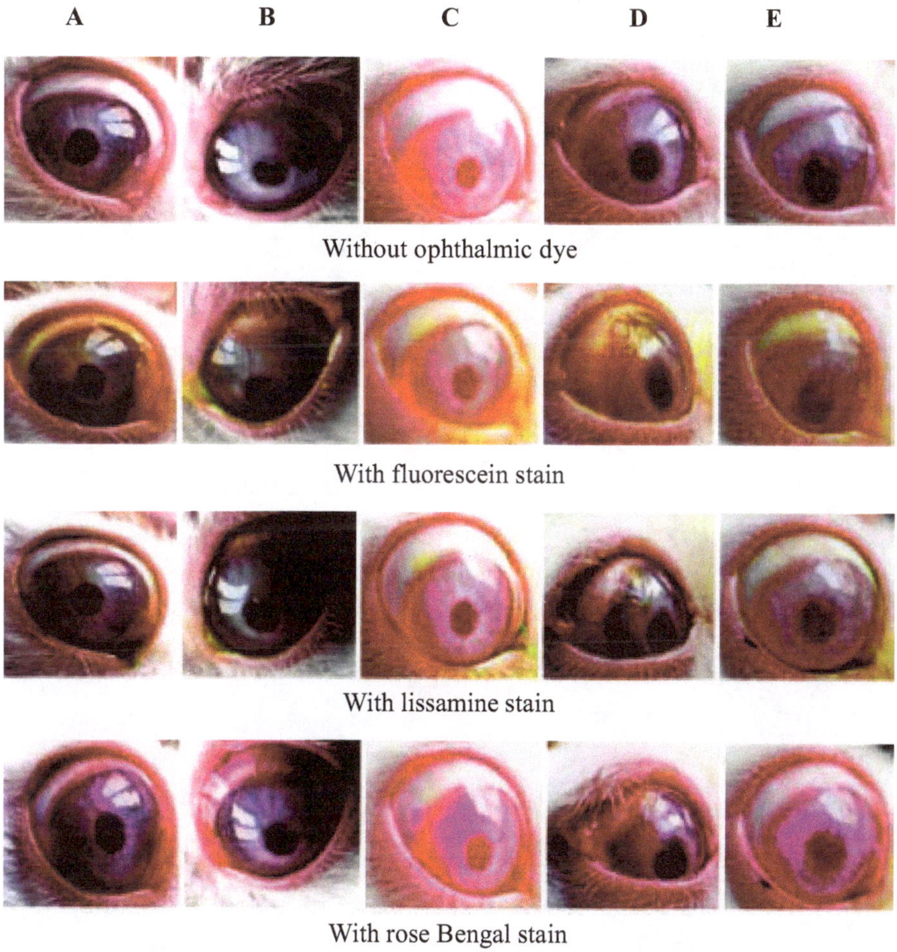

Colour photographs of treated groups on day 60 post implantation

10

Effect of PDGF-beta Gene Activated Acellular Matrix and Stem Cell Transplantation on Full Thickness Burn Wound in Rat Model

Full thickness burn wound will not heal spontaneously which need early excision and adequate coverage to prevent fluid loss and risk of infection. Major portion of the skin is lost during burn injury which is the active layer for protecting the entry of micro organism from outside environment. So far, meshed autologous skin graft is regarded as the gold standard for treating extensive full thickness burns. However, their frequent use may be hampered by several impediments such as limited availability, donor site morbidity, associated with additional scarring. Severe burn patients invariably lack additional skin donor site. Moreover, creation of donor site in burned patient is equivalent to second degree burn and which further increase the total body surface area affected (TBSA). In past decades, numerous biomaterials have been investigated for the use as a dermal skin substitute for burn patients but none give promising results. The innovative tissue engineered bioactive materials offer potential tissue regeneration and prevent the tissue deterioration.

The extracellular matrix (ECM) derived naturally from mammalian tissue have been successfully used as scaffold for tissue reconstruction and wound management in clinical applications. ECM can be derived from various tissue or organs of different species but most commonly, porcine small intestinal submucosa and urinary bladder have been successfully used as scaffold for reconstruction. ECM is obtained by process of decellularization that involves the use of various ionic and non ionic detergents, acids, enzymatic solutions and mechanical/physical methods. During the process of decellularization, parenchymal cells present in the tissues and non parenchymal cells those in the endothelial cells are removed. The remaining ECM preserves their native structural and functional proteins, glycoproteins and bioactive factors. These preserved bioactive factors having great potential for tissue repair and make the acellular matrix a very promising scaffold for tissue engineering. The natural matrices are easily infiltrated and remodeled by host cells into long lived functional tissue over the synthetic scaffold materials on implantation. Moreover, the structures of ECM obtained from xenogenic origin are easily conserved well by the different species lines without any adverse effects. The scaffold derived from urinary bladder matrix (UBM) only having intact basement membrane compares to other tissues and fundamentally changes healing by deployment of significant bioactive molecules. These biomolecules have the capacity to engage cells involved in natural wound healing, including progenitor cells that differentiate to fully functional adult cells in site specific tissues. The degradation of naturally occurring ECM has also been associated with release of growth factors, peptides and antibacterial activity many of which have been shown to maintain bioactivity.

The success of tissue engineering strategies, however, critically depends on the extent of blood vessel infiltration into the scaffolds. The primary function of vasculature is to facilitate the transport of nutrients and oxygen to cells invading from the host tissue and cells transplanted in the scaffolds. So far, a lot of efforts have been devoted to the stimulation of an angiogenic response, among which delivery of angiogenic factors such as basic fibroblast growth factor (bFGF), vascular endothelial growth factor (VEGF) and platelet-derived growth factor (PDGF) etc., have been widely employed. However, short half-life, protein instability, large dose required, the need for repeated administration and a high cost limit their application in practice. To overcome these limits, loading of functional genes has been evaluated as an alternative approach. DNA-incorporated matrices, the so-called gene activated matrices (GAMs), have been developed to act as depots for localized and sustained expression of the growth factors while simultaneously offering structural support and a matrix for new tissue deposition. So far GAMs have been employed to promote regeneration of several tissues such as bone, cartilage and skin.

Cutaneous wound healing requires a well-orchestrated integration of the complex biological and molecular events of cell migration and proliferation, as well as extracellular matrix deposition, angiogenesis and remodeling. Stem cells, due to their ability to differentiate into various tissue types by asymmetric replication, may create such a complex structure. Bone marrow-derived cells used in chronic wounds have been of particular interest. Bone marrow stromal cells are further found to synthesize higher amounts of collagen, FGF, and VEGF, when compare to native dermal fibroblasts, indicating a potential use in accelerating wound healing.

In this chapter, effect of gene embedded (pDNA-PDGF-BB) porcine acellular matrix with transfected mesenchymal stem cells on healing of full thickness burn in rat model is described.

Forty clinically healthy male Wistar rats are used in this study. The animals are anaesthetized with Xylazine at 5mg/kg and Ketamine HCl at 50mg/kg intra peritoneal. Before infliction of burn wound, the dorsal surface is shaved and sterilized with Povidone iodine. Contact burn is created by placing a heated custom-made steel bar (2 X 2 cm size) on the dorsum of the animal. Briefly, the bar is heated in flame at constant temperature of 130°C, placed on the dorsum of the animal for 30s at constant pressure. After infliction of burn wound, the animals is received intra-peritoneal injection of ringers lactate to resuscitate the fluid loss. To mimic the clinical situation, the necrosed tissue around the burn wound is excised to the level of the underlying muscular fascia 72 hrs after the injury, leaving the fascia intact. The average size of the resulting defects is 2 x2 cm full thickness burn wound.

Animals are randomly divided into five different groups consisting of 8 animals in each group and are treated according to the following table:

Group	Experimental model	Type of scaffold
Group A (control)	Full thickness burn wound	Silver sulfadiazine ointment
Group B	-do-	Porcine acellular urinary bladder (AUBM)
Group C	-do-	Porcine AUBM fabricated with pDNA-PDGF-B
Group D	-do-	Porcine AUBM seeded with rBMSC
Group E	-do-	Porcine AUBM fabricated with pDNA-PDGF-B along with rBMSC

The burn wound is replaced by the same size of the porcine AUBM. After filling the wound with the predefined material, the edge of the scaffold is sutured with surrounding skin layer with polyamide suture in interrupted pattern. To protect the burn wound from outside contamination and infection non adhesive pressure bandage is applied. Broad-spectrum antibiotic and anti-inflammatory drugs is mixed with drinking water and is given per orally for 5 days post operatively. Dressing of suture line with Povidone iodine is done after first week of surgery and in control group animals are dressed with silver sulfadiazine ointment. The efficacy of the porcine AUBM on reconstruction of full thickness burn wound defects is evaluated based on clinical observations, histopathological and colour digital imaging.

Preparation of Acellular Porcine Bladder: The porcine bladders samples is obtained from a local abattoir within 4 hrs of slaughter and transported to laboratory in a sterile ice cold contain phosphate buffer saline. The adhered fat, fascia of outside surface and residual urine in bladder lumen is completely removed. In luminal surface the urothelium and sub urothelium is removed surgically and remaining portion are subjected to incubation overnight in ice-cold hypotonic Tris buffer containing EDTA. After three washes with ice-cold PBS, the bladder is incubated for 24 h at 37°C with physical agitation in containing 1% Sodium dodecyl sulfate ionic detergent. After washing with detergents, the bladder sample is washed thrice with ice-cold PBS. Followed by, the bladder samples are transferred to the enzymatic solutions containing DNase, RNase, EDTA and Penicillin, in PBS 3hr at 37^{0}C with physical agitation to remove any remaining cellular material. Bladder is sterilized with ethanol for 3hrs and washed in PBS. Finally the biomaterials are stored in PBS at -20°C for further use and clinical trial.

Cloning of rat platelet derived growth factor-B on pVaxl vector and expression in stem cell: the process is beyond the objective and scope of this book. Briefly the process includes separation of rat peripheral blood monolayer cells, isolation of total RNA from PBMC, DNAse treatment of total RNA, preparation of complementary DNA, cloning of rat PDGF-B gene in pVAXI vector, amplification of rat PDGF-B from rat PBMCs, purification of amplified product, isolation of pVAXI plasmid, restriction enzyme digestion and ligation of vector and insert, preparation of E.coli competent cells by calcium chloride method, transformation of ligation in E.coli top 10 competent cells, screening of recombinant colonies, transfection of pVAXI-PDGF-B gene plasmid with rBMSC.

Collection of bone marrow, isolation, culture, colony forming assays, cell viability assay, flow cytometric analysis of CD markers, osteogenic differentiation, adipogenic differentiation, chondrogenic differentiation of rat bone marrow derived mesenchymal stem cell (rBMSC) is already described in detail in previous chapter of this book.

Fabrication of gene activated matrix: To facilitate the complete incorporation of pVAX1-PDGF-B complex into the porcine acellular matrix, the lipofectamine-pDNA polyplex complex is prepared. 75 μl of the solutions is added per side of the dried acellular matrix, which is kept in serum free media for 4 hrs. Then media is removed and complete media is added to the graft. Scaffold is then seeded with rBMSC on each side of the graft including a 15 min incubation time. Construct are cultured with growth media for transgenic expression study.

Clinical Observations: Feeding pattern and general behavioral changes is observed daily during the observation period. Rectal temperature, warmth of graft and adjoining area and exudation is recorded on days 0, 3, 5 and 7 postoperatively. Colour photographs and evaluation of wound closure is done on 0, 3, 7, 14, 21 and 28 days postoperatively and analyzed for healing status. The biopsy specimen is collected on 3, 7, 14, 21 and 28 post implantation days after euthanizing the animals for histopathological evaluation. The biopsy specimens are fixed in 10% Neutral Buffer Formalin (NBF). The implants are then processed for paraffin embedding technique to get thick paraffin section. The sections stain by hematoxylin and eosin to evaluate the healing process. The sections are observed under light microscope for epithelialization, inflammation, fibroplasia and neovascularization. The section is also subjected to Masson's Trichrome staining to observe the deposition of collagen. Indirect ELISA for antibody detection in rat serum in different post graft implant period is also done.

Result

On general observation, the animals are dull and have hunched back posture for first 24 hrs of post injury. After that animal is started to take feed partially and become normal by 3rd postoperative days. The rectal temperature and warmth of adjacent to the graft area is increased in the first 3 days in all groups and thereafter animal shows normal temperature. All the wounds appear apparently healthy throughout the observation period. As the wound healing is progressed, the area of wound reduces compare to initial wound size. Wound contraction and color digital photography confirm that group E and group D shows highest reduction in wound gap and compete healing is noticed on day 28, whereas, in other groups healing is not completed even after 28 days post injury. The enzyme linked immuno - sorbent assay reveal significant rise in antibody titer in all the groups from day 7 to day 21. Thereafter, significant reduction is noticed in all the groups. Group E shows significantly less antibody titer compared to all other groups at various intervals.

The biopsy specimens from the implantation site are collected on days 3, 7, 14, 21 and 28 post-implantation for the histopathological and RT-qPCR analysis. The result shows that neovasularization and collagen deposition is faster in group E compared to other groups. In early period, there is neovasularization and in later stage fully functional vessels are noticed. This is confirmed in both histopathological and gene expression studies. VEGF is produced in relatively high quantities with no significant differences between groups on day 7. On histological examination, more amounts of new vessel formation, fibroblast, and granulation tissue progression is noticed on group D and E compare to other groups. Increased production of PDGF-B gene simultaneously increase production of VEGF contributed in mural cell recruitment and new vessel formation. In gene expression study it is confirms that, there is increased expression of PDGF-B and VEGF in group D and E on day 14. The level of expression is significantly higher in group E then group D compare to all other groups. The fibroblast proliferation is much more in group D and E which indirectly increase the deposition extracellular matrix and collagen. This is confirmed on Masson's trichrome staining where deposition of new collagen is observed. On day 21, histological score is least in group E followed by group D. The epithelization is almost complete in both the groups and almost similar to the normal skin. In this study, it is observed that group E treated defects do not exhibit much wound contraction, suggesting that PDGF-B incorporated in the acellular scaffold may promote wound healing with minimal scar formation. On histological examination fully formed vasculature is noticed in group E compare to other groups. The result of RT-qPCR indicates that the group E exhibited the highest mRNA expression of VEGF, α-SMA and PDGF-B gradually increasing from weeks 1 to 4. On day 28, wound of groups E and D are completely covered with epidermis. The collagen fibers are best arranged and oriented parallel to the skin surface in group D and E suggesting a better healing of burn wound in these groups. All these results confirm that group E can resist the contraction, induce cell infiltration and neo-tissue formation, and promote blood vessel in-growth compare to all other groups. The expressions of PDGF-B, VEGF and ά-SMA genes are remained higher throughout the observation period, whereas in other groups these gene expressions are fluctuated and remain lowered. In conclusion, gene activated matrices along with stem cell can resist the contraction, induce earlier cell infiltration, neo-tissue formation, and promote blood vessel in-growth in burn wound. This study also establish the new biomaterial for delivery of therapeutic genes in full thickness burn wound healing and further facilitates the development of novel gene based biomaterial for tissue reconstruction. This study reports the first use of pVAX1-PDGF-B administration through acellular xenogeneic graft to promote full thickness burn wound healing.

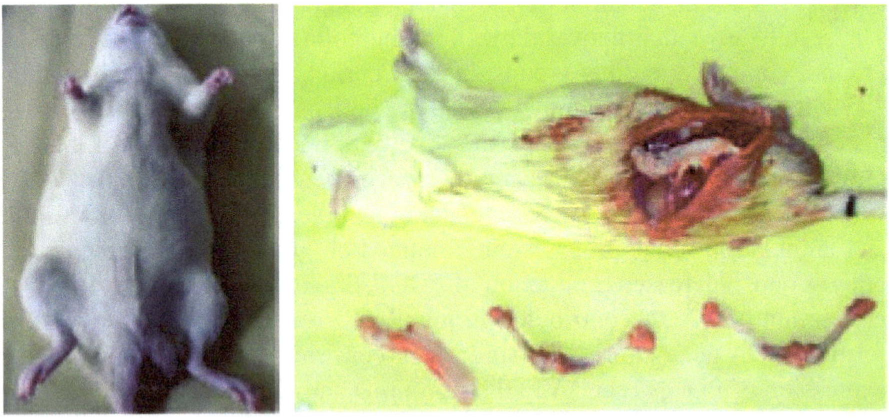

Collection of rat bone marrow from long bones

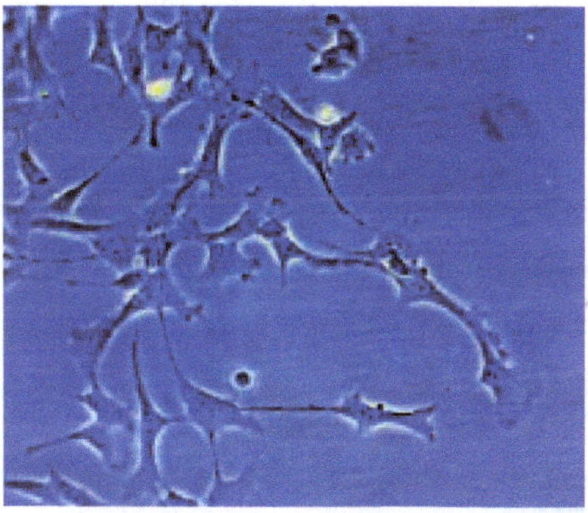

Rat bone marrow derived MSC

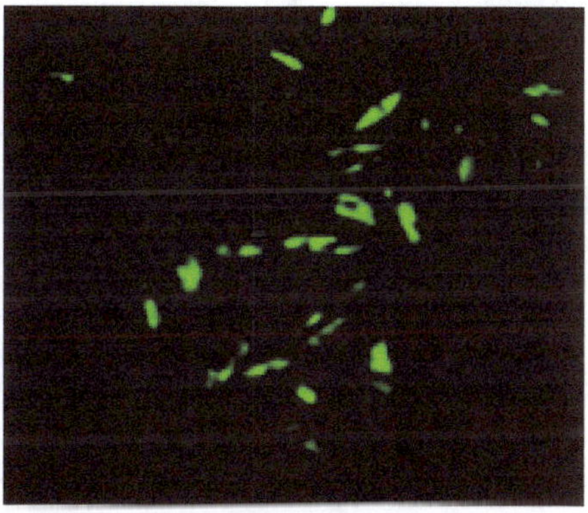

MSC characterized by surface marker STRO-1

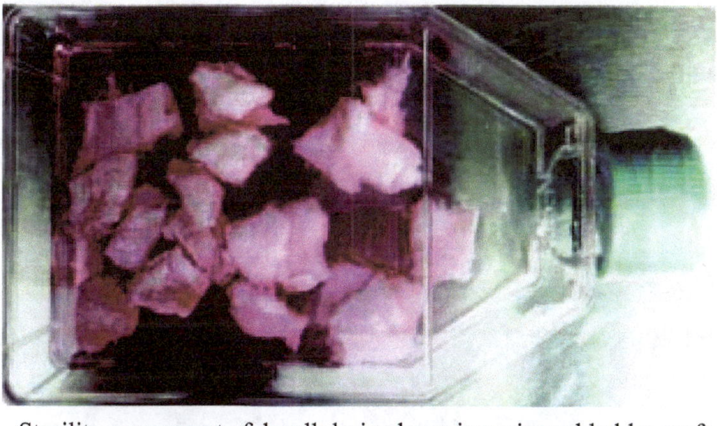

Sterility assessment of decellularized porcine urinary bladder graft

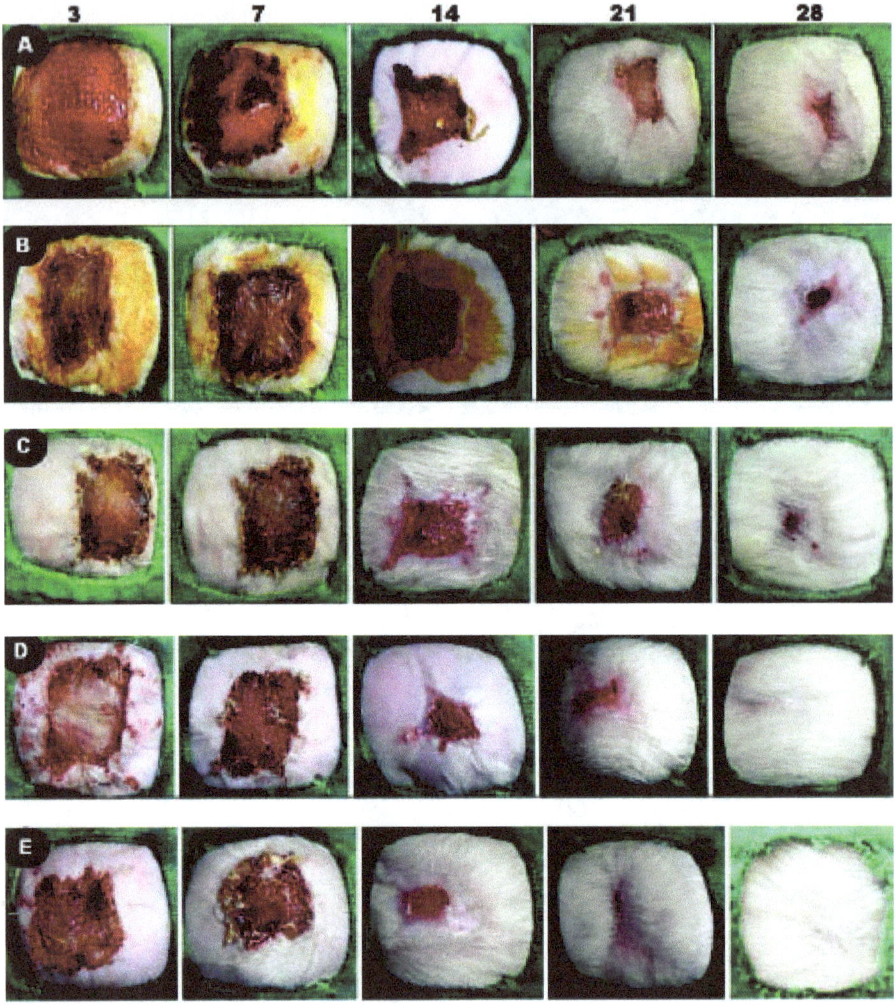

Digital photographs of healing of burn wounds in different groups in different intervals

11

Evaluation of Healing Potential of Chitosan and Porcine Small Intestinal Sub-Mucosa with Mesenchymal Stem Cells and Murine EGF for Full Thickness Burn Wound in Rat Model

Burn wounds are considered to be one of the most devastating kinds of trauma that affect the physical, physiological and psychological well being of an individual. Based on the depth of the affected area, burn wound is divided into three categories: first degree (superficial), second degree (partial) and third degree (full thickness). Extensive and deep burns result in scar formation and subsequent deformation of the affected part. Healing of burn wound involves several interrelated and overlapping stages such as inflammatory, proliferative and remodeling phases. The interaction of a variety of mediators, cells and extracellular matrix proteins are involved in this three phases of healing.

Burn wound therapy has been performed in various ways such as bioengineered skin grafts and administration of growth factors. Small intestinal sub-mucosa (SIS) is a resorbable xenogenic bioscaffold that has induced constructive remodeling in variety of animal models. It is unique from other acellular matrices as it contains few growth factors such as fibroblast growth factor (FGF) and transforming growth factor (TGF) that play a role in the regenerative process. Chitosan is currently proposed to be one of the most promising polymers in wound dressing development and it accelerates wound healing. Epidermal growth factor is known to stimulate growth of keratinocytes *in vitro*, thus it might be expected to promote wound healing.

In this chapter efficacy of Chitosan and porcine acellular small intestinal sub-mucosal (SIS) matrix seeded with bone marrow derived mesenchymal stem cells (BM-MSCs) and recombinant murine epidermal growth factor (m-EGF) on healing of full thickness burn wound in rat model is described.

Seventy clinically healthy adult Wistar rats of either sex are used in this study. The animals are anaesthetized with Xylazine at 5mg/kg and Ketamine HCL at 50mg/kg intra peritoneal. The animals are randomly divided into 7 groups A, B, C, D, E, F and G of ten animals each. In all the groups, a full thickness burn injury is created on the dorsum of each animal with a custom made iron bar of 2×2 cm size. The bar is heated in flame for 15 seconds and it is pressed on the surgically prepared dorsum of the animal with constant pressure for 10 seconds. Procedures are done under strict aseptic conditions. Treatment is performed according the following table:

Group	Experimental model	Type of scaffold
A	2x2 cm^2 full thickness burn wound	Silver sulfadiazine
B	-do-	Medical grade chitosan
C	-do-	Chitosan +rMSC
D	-do-	Chitosan + rMSC +mEGF
E	-do-	Decellularized porcine SIS
F	-do-	r-MSC seeded porcine SIS
G	-do-	r-MSC seeded porcine SIS +mEGF

Recombinant murine EGF (Sigma) is used at a dose of 1 μg/wound continuously for 5 days. Third passage bone marrow derived mesenchymal stem cells are injected at the wound margin at a dose rate of 1×10^6 cells continuously for 5 days. Antibiotic (Cephalexin @ 10 mg/ kg body weight) and anti-inflammatory (Meloxicam @ 0.05 mg/kg body weight) drugs are given orally for 5 days postoperatively. The efficacy of Chitosan and the acellular scaffolds with r-MSC and m-EGF for the repair of full-thickness burn injury is evaluated based on different parameters. The animals are observed for the evidence of cutaneous healing by serial subjective evaluation of wound on 7, 14, 21 and 28 days postoperatively. After euthanizing two animals of each group on 7, 14, 21, and 28 days the burn wound healing is evaluated by clinical, histopathological, immunological, immunohistochemical and matrix metalloproteinase marker studies.

Porcine small intestine is collected aseptically from local abattoir and sub mucosa is separated. Obtained SIS is subjected to 1% SDS ionic detergent for decellularization. After 12h complete removal of cellular and nuclear element is revealed by histology and scanning electron microscopy. When compared to native SIS only negligible quantity of DNA could be detected by DNA quantification.

Collection of bone marrow, isolation, culture, colony forming assays, cell viability assay, flow cytometric analysis of CD markers, osteogenic differentiation, adipogenic differentiation, chondrogenic differentiation of rat bone marrow derived mesenchymal stem cell (rMSC) is already described in detail in previous chapter of this book.

Acellular SIS matrix is seeded with third passage of rMSC and it is kept in humidified atmosphere with 5%CO_2 at 37^{0}C for 7 days. Histology and scanning electron microscopy is confirmed the attachment of rMSC on the surface of scaffold.

Clinical Observations: Feeding pattern and general behavioral changes is observed daily during the observation period. Rectal temperature, warmth of graft and adjoining area and exudation is recorded on days 0, 3, 5 and 7 postoperatively. Colour photographs and evaluation of wound closure is done on 0, 3, 7, 14, 21 and 28 days postoperatively and analyzed for healing status. The biopsy specimen is collected on 3, 7, 14, 21 and 28 post implantation days after euthanizing the animals for histopathological evaluation. The biopsy specimens are fixed in 10% Neutral Buffer Formalin (NBF). The implants are then processed for paraffin embedding technique to get thick paraffin section. The sections stain by hematoxylin and eosin to evaluate the healing process. The sections are observed under light microscope for epithelialisation, inflammation, fibroplasia and neovascularization. The section is also subjected to Masson's Trichrome staining to observe the deposition of collagen. Indirect ELISA for antibody detection in rat serum in different post graft implant period is also done.

Result

On general observation, the animals are dull and have hunched back posture for first 24 hrs of post injury. After that animal is started to take feed partially and become normal by 3rd postoperative days. Rectal temperature and body weight is reduced in animals of all groups when compared with pre-burn day. Wound warmth and wound exudation is increased in Chitosan treated groups (B, C, D) during initial days of this study. In control group (A), wound appeared is to be necrosed during initial days. Later on, it's sloughed off and granulation tissue formation is started. In Chitosan treated group (B, C &D) there are expansion in the wound size after debridement. Graft initially is appeared pale which later on is vascularized. Wound contraction and digital photography shows good healing reduction of wound size progressively is reduced in groups C, D, F and G.

Enzyme linked immune sorbent assay and lymphocyte stimulation test reveal increased antibody titer in group E. In stem cell and growth factor treated groups, there is reduction in immune response.

Histopathologically, on day 7, there is complete destruction of epidermis in all the groups. Necrotic material and inflammatory exudates are present in all treatment groups. Infiltration of polymorphonuclear cells into the dermis is noticed. Necrotic material and inflammatory exudates are present in all the groups. There are patchy hemorrhages at various points. Masson trichrome staining is also demonstrate the presence of fibrin clots and exudates. On day 14, presence of inflammatory cells is found. Necrotic materials and exudates are absent. Continuity of epidermis is established in all the implanted groups whereas it is only partially established in rest of the groups but there is thickening of epidermis. Neovascularization is evident in all the groups. Collagen fibers are thin and densely packed as observed in Masson trichrome staining. On day 21, number of inflammatory cells is less as compared to day 14. Epithelial continuity is established in all the groups. Epidermal thickening is comparatively less when compared to day 14. Fibroblasts are present in large numbers. Extend of inflammation has reduced. There are neovascularization in all the treatment groups. In Masson's trichrome staining collagen fibers are thin and densely packed. Sweat glands are started appearing in group E. On day 28, epidermis has come to its normal appearance. Inflammation is present only at the level of dermis. Number of fibroblast is less as compared to day 21. In groups E, D, F and G, presence of hair follicles, sweat gland and sebaceous glands is seen. In Masson's trichrome staining collagen fibers are appeared to be thin but packed so closely as compared to the normal rat skin. In short, histopathological scoring of biopsy specimen reveal a better positive scoring and collagen fiber arrangement in group G, where the burn wound is treated with seeded SIS, rMSC and mEGF. In stem cell and growth factor treated Chitosan groups also good healing is recorded. In group G, higher expression of MMP-2 is indicating the activity of mEGF in the wound healing. In other groups no MMPs are expressed. In conclusion: acellular SIS matrix is found to have good healing potential for full thickness skin burn wound; Chitosan is not as effective as SIS matrix in providing coverage for full thickness burn wound; Chitosan in combination with rMSC and mEGF is proved to be efficient for full thickness burn wound healing and when combined with rMSC and mEGF acellular SIS matrix is accelerated healing of full thickness skin burn wound.

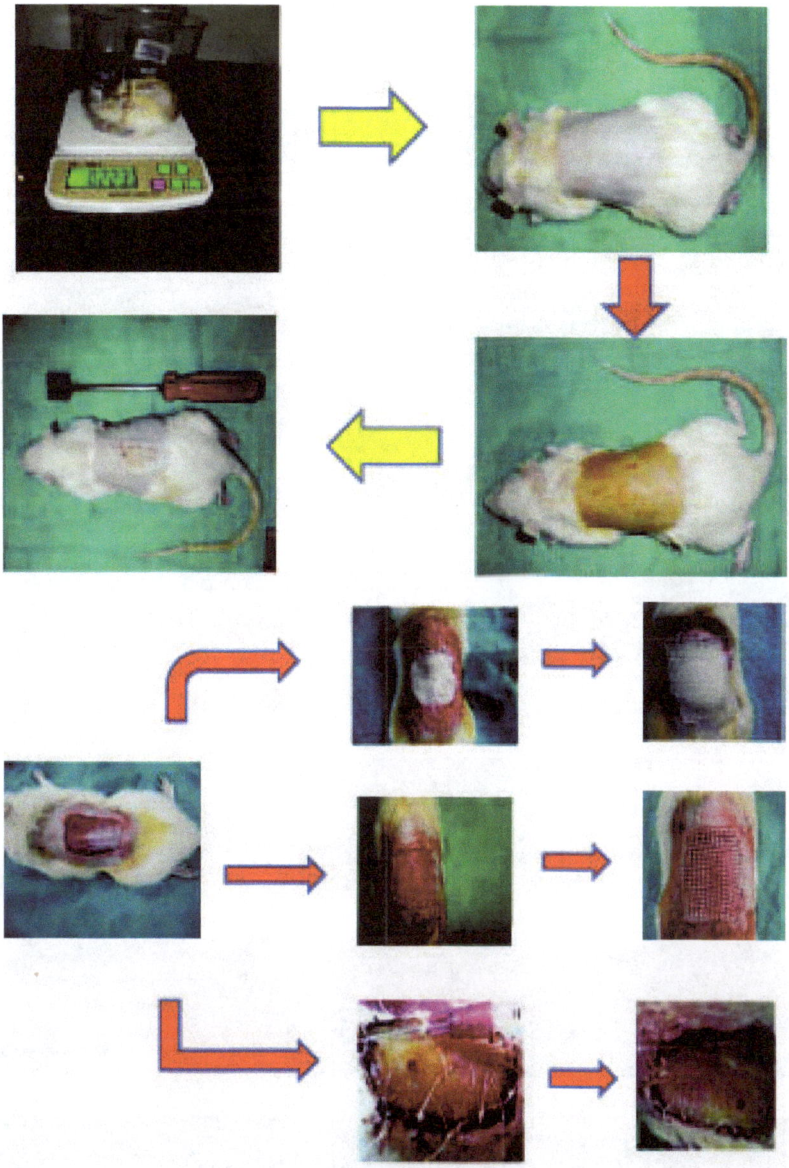

Creation of burn wound on the dorsum and application of chitosan, acellular SIS and injection of rMSC/mEGF at the margin of burn wound.

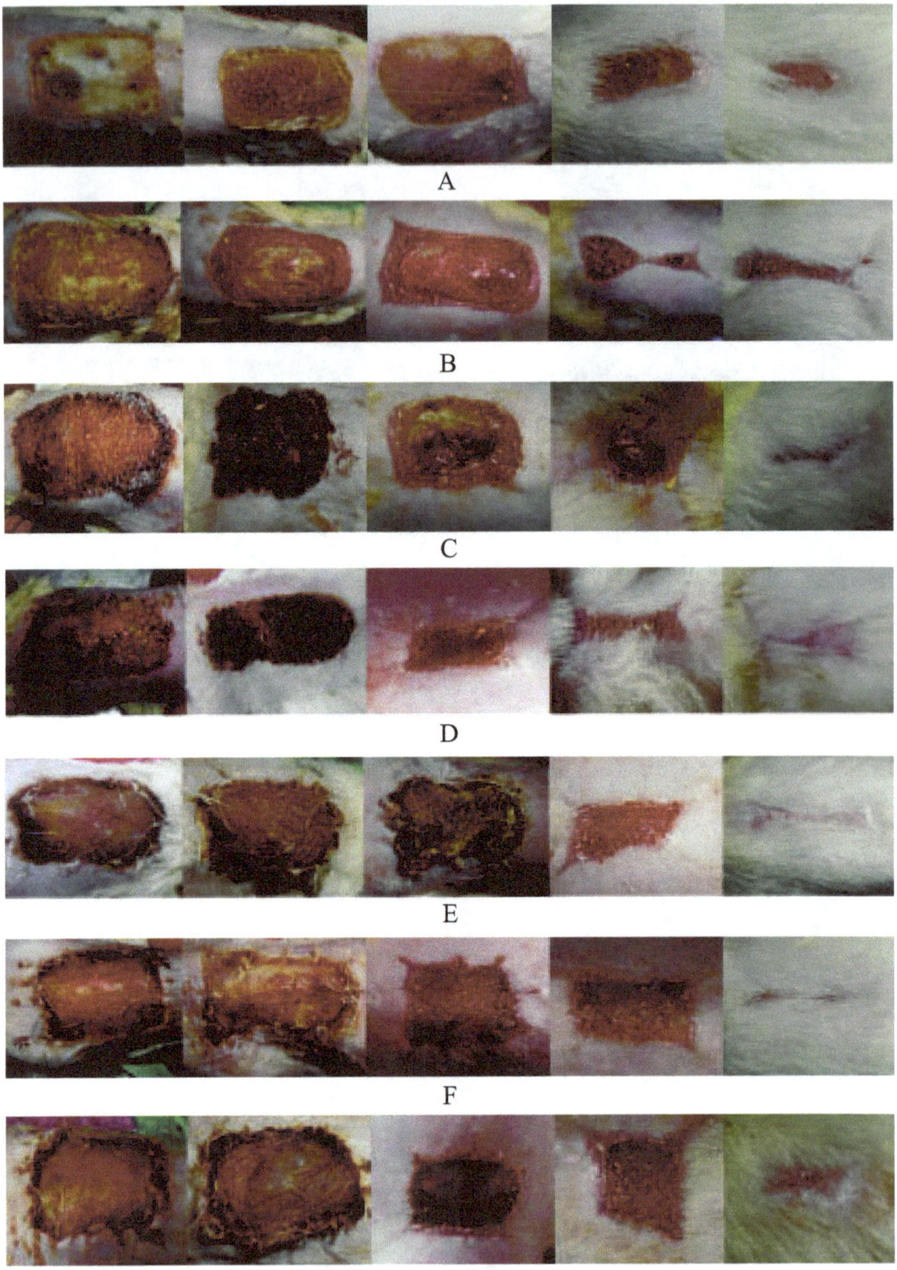

G

DAY 3 DAY 7 DAY 14 DAY 21 DAY 28

Computerized planimetry /colour digital imaging in different groups in different intervals

12

Evaluation of Mesenchymal Stem Cells with Conditioned Media and m-EGF for Regeneration of Liver Tissue after Partial Hepatectomy in Rats

The liver is an organ that plays a central role in maintaining metabolic homeostasis, in its functions of metabolism, synthesis and storage of nutrients. The cells in the liver are parenchyma cells and non- parenchyma cells. The former include hepatocytes (80% of the cell population) and the later includes endothelial cells, Kupffer cells, lymphocytes and stellate cells. Liver dysfunction or failures are having different etiologies. Liver cancer has the fifth highest cancer incidence in the world, and is the third highest cause of cancer related deaths, with resection of the liver remaining the only curative option.

Following liver injury, the repair process involves two distinct phases: a regenerative phase, in which injured liver cells are replaced with regenerated hepatocytes; and a phase known as fibroplasia or fibrosis, in which connective tissue replace normal parenchyma tissue. The process even though initially beneficial becomes pathogenic when it is not controlled appropriately. Extensive accumulation of extra-cellular matrix (ECM) components ultimately leads to cirrhosis and liver failure. Thus, the ideal strategy to treat liver injury is to generate new hepatocytes replacing damaged cells without causing excessive ECM deposition.

Hepatic resections are both associated with, and dependent on a rapid proliferation and regeneration of the remnant liver. But many patients experience temporary or permanent hepatic insufficiency after surgery, usually because they have factors potentially limiting liver regeneration, such as advanced age, steatosis, and liver cirrhosis. Therefore, it is essential to optimize liver regenerative capacity in patients with suboptimal liver function or who are scheduled to undergo major hepatectomy. Exploring the newer scientific discoveries governing liver regeneration could contribute to enlightening our understanding of the mechanisms behind this process. This could offer new treatment strategies, not only to patients with advanced liver cancer, but also to patients suffering from acute and chronic liver failure, as the liver is the major detoxifying organ of the body and is likely to be injured by ingested toxins.

Orthotropic liver transplantation is a life-saving treatment for patients with end-stage liver disease, but it is limited by organ shortages, high expense, graft rejection, and the requirement for long-term immunosuppression and considerable long-term side effects that include chronic renal failure, post transplant lymphoproliferative disease, and cardiovascular complications.

The search for new therapies has been actively pursued for several decades, primarily in the form of artificial liver support devices and hepatocytes transplantation, yet both of these modalities remain experimental. During tissue injury, it has been suggested that bone marrow stem cells are mobilized and migrate to the injured organ to maintain physiologic homeostasis. This theory has formed the basis for regenerative therapy whereby treatment with appropriate stem cells might ameliorate specific diseases. It has been mentioned that MSCs can move toward areas of injury in response to signals of cellular damage, which are known as homing signals. This migration property of MSCs is important in regenerative medicine because various parenteral routes can be used depending on the damaged tissue or organ. MSCs can be transplanted into the liver by intravenous, intraperitoneal, intrahepatic, intrasplenic, or portal-venous injection, however there effects have differed based on their injection routes.

The secretome or conditioned media is defined as the richly complex set of molecules secreted by stem cells or shed from their surface. The idea of using stem cell secretome or conditioned media is based on the concept that the secretome is responsible for a considerable portion of the therapeutic potential of stem cells. The MSC secretome contains a large number of growth factors and cytokines that are critical for the repair of injured tissues. Since paracrine factors released by stem cells can accumulate in the CM, it can be utilized as a cell-free therapy.

EGF is a polypeptide produced in the submandibular glands, Brunner's glands and kidneys. It stimulates growth of many cells including liver parenchyma cells both *in vivo* and *in vitro* and it is expressed under normal physiological conditions in the adult liver, and gets markedly up regulated during the process of regeneration after liver injury or partial hepatectomy. The administration of EGF accelerates the proliferation of hepatocytes, regardless of what recombinant protein or gene therapy strategy is used.

In this chapter the potential of mesenchymal stem cells, conditioned media and epidermal growth factor in promoting liver regeneration is compared following partial hepatectomy in rat model.

Eighty Wistar rats of either sex are used in this study and randomly divided into 8 groups, *viz.*, group A to H of 10 animals each. Animals of each group are given treatment according to the following table.

Group	Treatment
A	Phosphate buffered saline (Control)
B	Conditioned media (CM)
C	Rat bone marrow derived mesenchymal stem cells (r-BMSC)
D	Murine Epidermal growth factor (m-EGF)
E	CM + m-EGF
F	rBMSC + CM
G	rBMSC + m-EGF
H	rBMSC + m-EGF +CM

The animals are given stem cells (1.5×10^6, I/V), conditioned media (0.5ml, I/V), m-EGF (9µg, S/C) at three different intervals. The animals are sacrificed on 10th, 20th, 30th, 40th day and liver samples are collected for histopathology and immunohistochemistry. The blood samples are also collected for biochemical analysis. Clinico-physiological parameters are also recorded.

Collection of bone marrow, isolation, culture, colony forming assays, cell viability assay, flow cytometric analysis of CD markers, osteogenic differentiation, adipogenic differentiation, chondrogenic differentiation of rat bone marrow derived mesenchymal stem cell (rMSC) is already described in detail in previous chapter of this book.

The rats are anaesthetized with Midazolam @5mg/kg and Ketamine @50mg/kg intravenously. The cranio-ventral abdomen of the rats are shaved and sterilized with 5% povidone iodine. The rats are restrained in dorsal recumbency. A midline incision is made from the xiphoid cartilage to umbilicus and cranial abdomen is exposed. The liver is exteriorized and three knot technique is used at the base of lateral and median lobe of the liver. Then respective lobes are resected (65-70% of total size) after proper ligation. Bleeding is checked and abdomen and skin are sutured in routine fashion in layers. The animals are given postoperatively antibiotic and anti-inflammatory drugs for three days.

Clinico-physiological parameters like rectal temperature are recorded on the day of surgery and for five days continuously postoperatively. Body weight are observed and recorded on 10th, 20th, 30th, and 40th days in all experimental groups.

Two ml of blood is collected from orbital plexus of rats for estimation of ALT, AST, ALP, Albumin, Total protein, Bilirubin, GGT using standard commercially available kits. Blood glucose is estimated in the blood collected from tip of the tail using glucometer. One ml of blood is used for hemoglobin and PCV estimation on 10th, 20th, 30th and 40th days post surgery.

Regeneration coefficient is used for quantitative evaluation of the regeneration processes.

Matrix metalloproteinase-9 (MMP-9) is estimated by using ELISA kit on 10th, 20th, 30th and 40th days postoperatively. Tissue inhibitors of matrix metalloproteinases-2 (TIMP-2) are estimated using Rat TIMP-2 ELISA kit on 10th, 20th, 30th and 40th days post-operatively.

Liver tissues are collected on 10th, 20th, 30th and 40th day's interval for histological evaluation. Liver specimens are fixed in 10% neutral buffered formalin. The samples are then processed for paraffin embedding technique to get 5 micron thick paraffin section. The section is stained by Hematoxylin-Eosin (HE) to evaluate the regeneration process of liver tissue. Sections are also stained with Masson's Trichrome for demonstration of collagen deposition in regenerated liver tissue at different intervals of experiment.

For immunohistochemical studies, two hours before sacrifice, rats are administered BrdU intraperitoneal. After being anesthetized, liver tissues are removed and fixed with 10% neutral buffered formalin (NBF) for overnight, and then the tissues are shifted to fresh 10% NBF. Tissue sections are prepared and coated slides are used.

Result

The biochemical parameters ALT, AST, ALP, GGT, bilirubin, total protein, albumin and blood glucose are determined at different intervals. In group A there is significant elevation in transaminase, ALP, GGT, bilirubin indicating that the liver damage is not restored properly. Similarly there is decline in total protein, albumin and glucose in group A showing that the remnant liver is not able to restore its function back. However, group H and G shows normal range of values of ALT, AST, GGT, bilirubin, total protein, albumin and blood glucose. While other groups B, C, D, E, F are better than group A, but not well enough as group G and H. The parameters like haemoglobin, PCV, rectal temperature remain more or less in normal range in all groups. Body weight declined initially but later on increased in all the groups, however, there are significant decrease in body weight in group A. Regeneration coefficient calculated based on liver weight is higher in groups H and G in comparison to group A. The matrix metalloproteinase level has significantly increased in all groups compare to their base value except in group A and B. The MMP-9 value is significantly higher in group H followed by that in group G, F, C, E, D, B, A in the descending order. Whereas TIMP-2 is significantly higher in groups A, B compare to all other groups. On day 40, TIMP-2 concentration is significantly highest in groups A followed by in group B and C. However, the TIMP-2 concentration is significantly lowest in group H followed by group G, F, E, D in ascending order.

Colour digital imaging in group A reveals that size of the liver as such do not increase much on day 10 while subsequently hypertrophy is observed in other lobes but livers comparatively paler in appearance. In groups B, C, D and E liver size progressively increase from day 20 onwards and texture of liver also improve. In group F, on day 40, the liver size is enlarged, normal texture and contours almost established. In group G and H, hypertrophy and liver enlargement is noticed from day 10 onwards and on day 40, liver colour, texture, size and contour is established as like normal.

Histopathological examination in group A on day 30 reveals fibroblast proliferation, neovascularization, newly formed hepatocytes. On day 40, newly formed hepatocytes can be seen; enlarged cells with hyperchromatic nuclei and vacuolation are observed. In group B, on day 40 there is bile duct proliferation along with more number of Kupffer cells in the regenerated area, no distinct boundary of hepatocytes. In group C, on day 40 newly formed hepatocytes, bile pigment deposition is seen, however, sinusoidal arrangement is not properly formed. In group D and E, on day 30, newly formed hepatocytes with normal nucleus, elongated Kupffer cells are seen. On day 40, bile duct proliferation, bile pigment deposition and newly formed hepatocytes with normal nucleus seen. In group F, on day 40, newly formed hepatocytes with homogenous cytoplasm and normal nuclei and bile duct proliferation in the regenerated area is noticed. In group G, on day 30, bile duct proliferation, nucleus of newly formed hepatocytes with no proper cell boundaries is seen. On day 40, regenerated areas with properly formed hepatocytes can be seen. In group H, on day 30, neovascularization, more number of Kupffer cells in the area can be seen. On day 40, dividing hepatocytes, lymphocyte infiltration and newly formed hepatocytes are noticed. In a short, maximum degenerative changes are noticed in group A followed by group B, C and D. The group H has the least number of degenerative changes.

Masson's trichrome staining in liver section of group A reveals collagen deposition in between the newly formed hepatocytes and around the proliferated bile duct which was subsequently increased from day 10 onwards up to day 40. In group B, fibroblast proliferation in between the hepatocytes got reduced and more organised. In group C, the fibrous tissue proliferation is limited around the bile ducts and at the junction of regeneration. In groups D, E and F, the fibrous tissue deposition is less and more organised. In group G, the extracellular deposition at the regenerated site is decreased from day 10 to day 40. In group H, the fibroblast proliferation and extracellular matrix deposition get significantly reduced on day 30 and it get more organized. In a short, maximum collagen deposition is seen in group A followed by in group B and C.

Immunohistochemistry is performed to evaluate the uptake of BrdU by the regenerated cells. It is observed that maximum BrdU stained nuclei is observed in group H followed by group G on day 40, whereas, it is very less in group A. The BrdU stained cells are higher in number in groups in which stem cell give alone or in combined with growth factor EGF. Tracing of transplanted mesenchymal stem cells are done using DAPI. It is a fluorescent dye that gives blue fluorescence and it binds to AT rich region of DNA.

In conclusion, partial hepatectomy model with surgical removal of 65-70% liver lobe is standardized and successfully used in this study. Rat bone marrow derived mesenchymal stem cells are found to induce hepatocytes proliferation; whereas, EGF induces more angiogenesis. Conditioned media is not as effective as stem cell and EGF. Rat bone marrow derived mesenchymal stem cells combined with EGF and conditioned media promotes a higher level of liver regeneration and reduces extracellular matrix deposition in hepatectomised model.

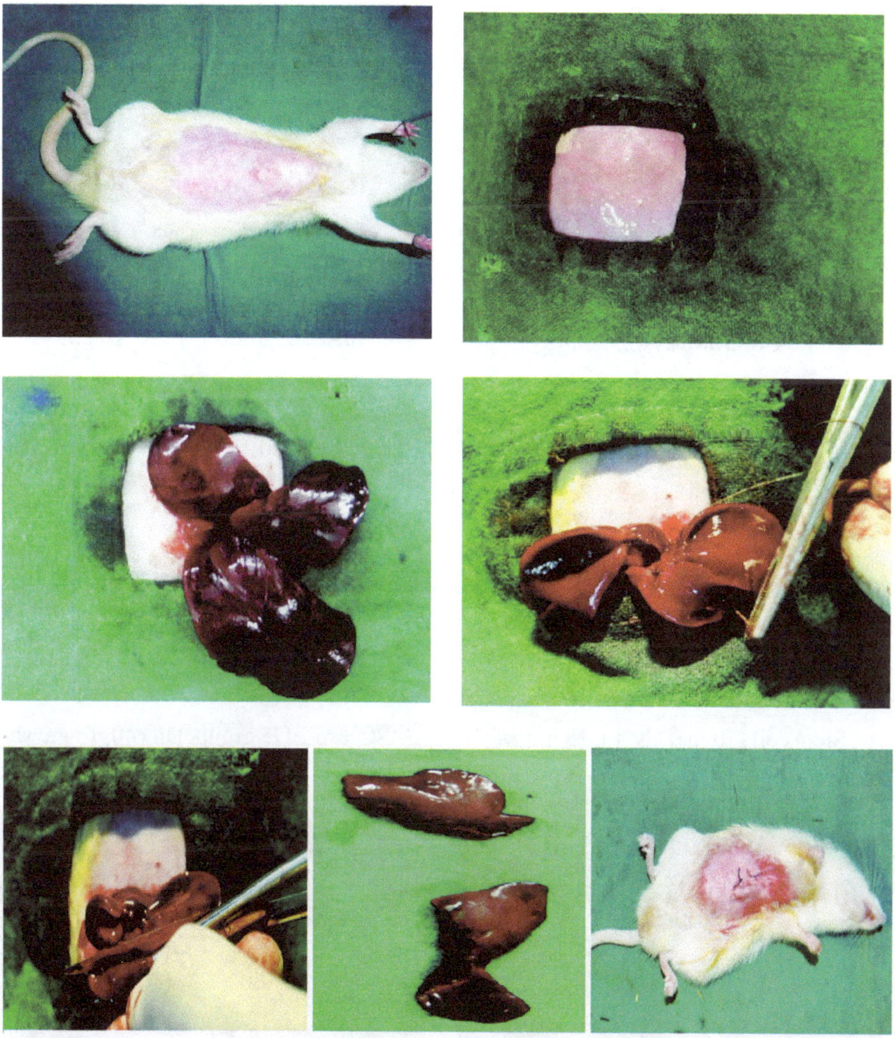

Exteriorized left lateral and medial liver lobe under general anesthesia, resection of these lobes and then ligated the liver stump with catgut

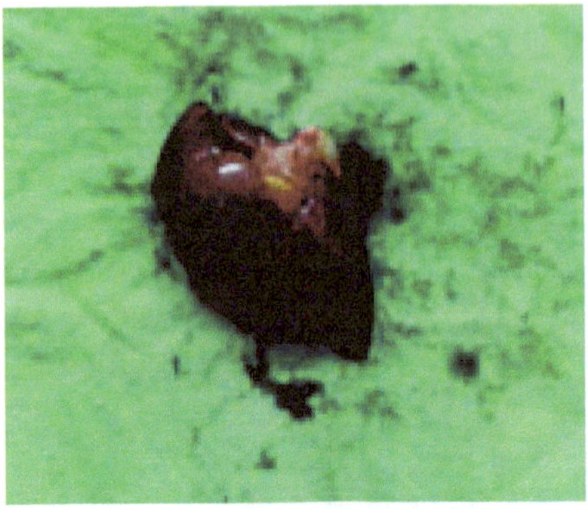

Control-Day 40, 7gm

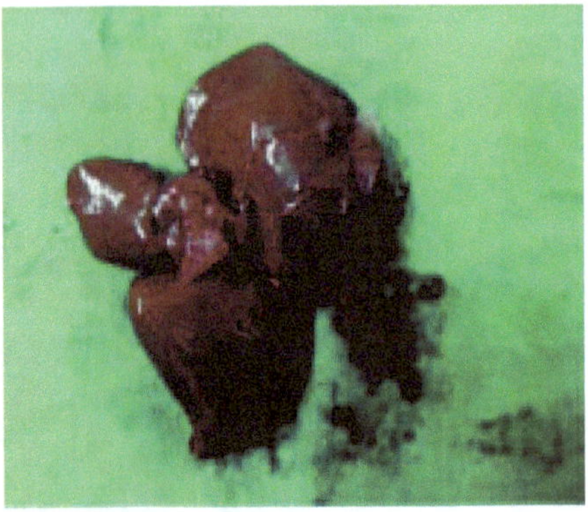

m-EGF group-Day 40, 10 gm

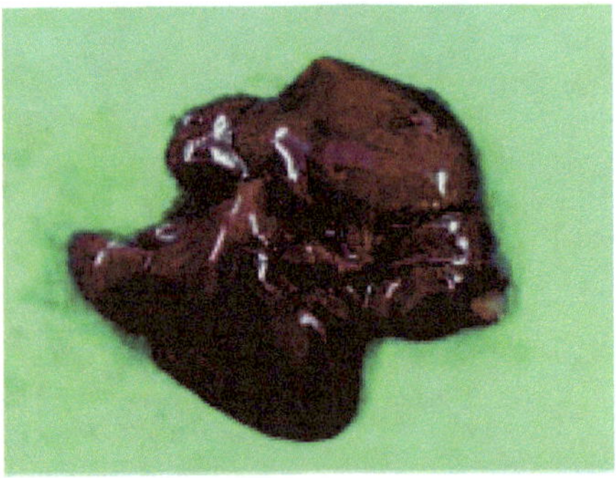

Stem cell group, Day 40, 13 gm wt

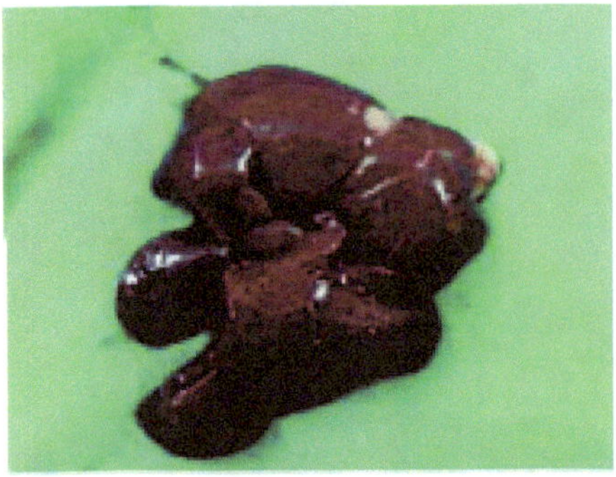

MSC + m-EGF group, Day 40, 15 gm wt

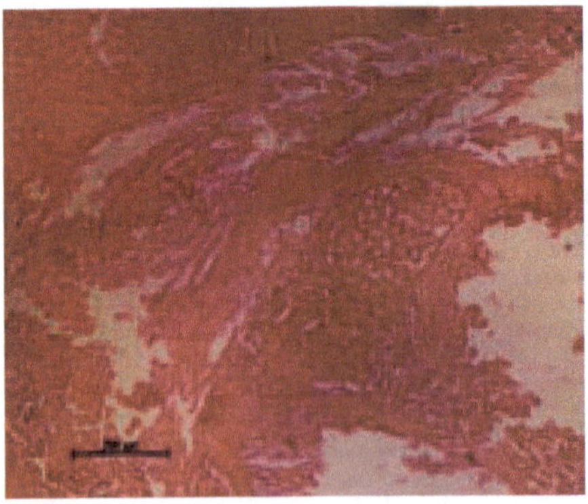

Control: Extensive collagen deposition, absence of normal liver cell parenchyma

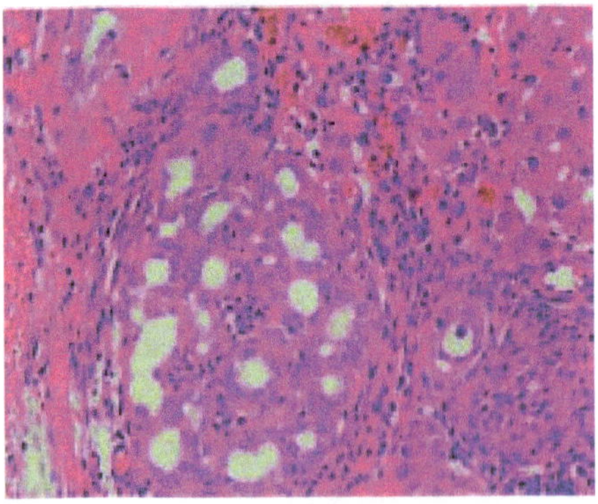

MSC: Normal liver cell parenchyma, very less collagen deposition at the junction, regeneration of new hepatocytes around new portal triad.

13

Role of Embryonic Stem cell (ESC)-Hydroxyapatite Construct with Growth Proteins for Osteogenesis in the Repair of Bone Defects in Rabbit Model

Bone is the only tissue in the body able to heal without microscopical scarring. On the other hand fracture healing is a slow process causing long immobilization periods with consequently high costs for fracture healing giving rise to delayed healing, fibrous healing or non-healing with subsequent problems for both, the patient and the orthopedic surgeon. Fracture healing is complex phenomenon which involves numerous cells, regulators of cell function and biochemical interactions in the repair process. The healing potential of bone, in a fracture model is influenced by a variety of biochemical, biomechanical, cellular, hormonal and pathological mechanisms. A continuous occurring state of bone deposition, resorption and remodeling facilitates the healing process.

Biodegradable and bioinert ceramic materials such as hydroxyapatite (HA), tri-calcium phosphate (TCP), aluminum-calcium-phosphate (ALCAP) ceramics provides scaffold to support the attachment and migration of newly formed bone cells into the osseous defect and also help in formation of a vascular network through the newly formed bone. Bioceramic also act as a carrier to deliver stem cells for osteogenesis.

Specific bone-inductive proteins/growth factors can induce bone formation and healing *in vivo*. These morphogens are therefore, to be an ideal alternative to autogenous bone grafts. These findings initiating intensive research into bone regeneration orchestrated by putative soluble signals and lead to the discovery and identification of an entirely novel family of protein initiators collectively called the bone morphogenic protein (BMPs), which belong to transforming growth factors-ß (TGF- ß) super family. These growth factors might possess a biological activity that is site and tissue specific in the induction of bone formation. Different growth factors have been demonstrated to possess osteoinductive and fracture healing properties.

Stem cells have therapeutic potential in the realm of orthopaedic surgery because of their capacity to self-renew and differentiate into various types of mature cells and tissues, including bone. Embryonic stem cells (ESCs) are pluripotent cells derived from the inner cell mass of pre-implantation embryos and represent embryonic precursor cells that give rise to any cell type in the embryo. Specifically, it has been shown that ES cells can differentiate into osteogenic cells under selective culture conditions. These osteogenic cells are capable of *in vitro* producing bone nodules in three dimensional scaffolds.

The potentials for using osteogenic stem cells in orthopaedic for bone and cartilage defect healing is immense, and is likely to further expand significantly in future. These approaches have included the implantation of osteoconductive extracellular matrix scaffold and the implantation of bone morphogenic proteins in various matrices. The most novel approach for this purpose is to combine a scaffold-matrix, living cells and biologically active molecules or factors together to form a tissue engineered construct (TEC) to promote the repair and regeneration of bony tissue.

In this chapter, the potential of cultured allogenic embryonic stem cells seeded in a calcium hydroxyapatite (HA/TCP) bioscaffold to generate new bone formation in a segmental bone defect with or without growth factors in rabbit model is described.

The study is conducted in 36 male adult New Zealand White rabbits divided into six equal groups. The groups and treatment on each group are as follows:

Group	Treatment
A	Empty defect (Control)
B	Defect filled with HA-TCP bioceramic
C	rESC with HA-TCP bioceramic
D	rESC with HA-TCP bioceramic + BMP-2
E	rESC with HA-TCP bioceramic + TGF-ß1
F	rESC with HA-TCP bioceramic + IGF-1

A biphasic composite bioceramic (calcium hydroxyapatite and tricalcium phosphate) namely HA-TCP with elements in the following percentage: calcium hydroxyapatite-65% and tricalcium phosphate 35%, and porosity of 200–450 µm is used as sterile ceramic granules.

Isolation of rabbit embryonic stem cells

Embryo recovery and collection: Each female rabbit is injected with PMSG intramuscularly in normal saline. After 72 hours of first injection, female rabbits are injected with HCG intravenously. Female rabbits are mated naturally.

Collection of embryos is done by flushing the uterine horns and oviducts of rabbits 84-96 hours after mating. Embryos are collected at blastocyst stage by flushing the uterine horn with modified phosphate buffered saline.

Derivation of ES Cells: The embryos collected are seeded on buffalo fetal fibroblast feeder layers. In this technique whole embryo, with its zona pellucida are plated on a mitomycin-C treated feeder layer. Two days after plating, the attachment of the whole embryo to the feeder layer is observed and the medium replaced with fresh medium on a daily basis. The trophoectoderm layer began to expand on the 2-3 day of culturing. The inner cell mass (ICM) like cells is formed dome structure. The cells are then incubated at 37°C in a humified 5% carbon dioxide environment in a CO_2 incubator. Once confluence, cells are passaged 2-3 times to increase the cell population. After ES cells population is established, it is then confirmed by characterization with different markers by alkaline phosphatase staining and immuno cytochemistry.

Preparation of fibroblast monolayer, collection of fetus, isolation of fetal skin fibroblast cells, setting of monolayer of fibroblast cells of fetal skin and sub culture is described in detail in published paper: Bhadane *et al* (2018).

All the animals are operated under general anaesthesia with xylazine hydrochloride and ketamine hydrochloride and strict surgical asepsis, a unilaterally 5mm bone defects are created in the radial diaphysis. A 2 cm medial incision over the radius is given, soft tissue is dissected and the bone is exposed by gentle retraction of the muscles. A Hohmann retractor is placed between ulna and radius to protect the ulna. A 5mm segmental osteo-periosteal diaphyseal defect is created with an oscillating bone saw that is continuously cooled by irrigation with 0.9% sterile cold saline solution. The periosteum is removed with the bone and 5mm of periosteum is stripped from each side of the remaining radius. The bone gap is irrigated with sterile physiological saline solution and ceramic granules (or nothing) fitted into the gap as per treatment protocol for different groups. Muscles, fascia and skin are separately closed over the defect with resorbable sutures. A wooden splint with bandage is applied on the test bone for one week.

All the animals are kept in isolated cages and administered with broad spectrum antibiotic for 5 consecutive days. The analgesic is administered for 3 days. The wound is dressed until the complete healing of the incision is seen and sutures are removed. The animals are observed for the evidence of wound healing, radiographic bone healing postoperatively and they are euthanized for the study of gross morphology, histology, and scanning electron microscopy on 40th postoperative day. Medio-lateral and anterio-posterior radiographs are taken immediately after implantation and subsequently on days 7, 15, 30, and 40th postoperative day

Result

Superovulation is successfully achieved in female New Zealand rabbits following injection of PMSG-HCG protocol followed by natural mating. A very good quality and good numbers of embryos are collected by flushing the uterine horns and oviducts of rabbits after 84-96 hours of mating.

The medium is used for culture and derivation of the stem cells consisted of Knockout Dulbecco's modified Eagle's medium with 5% FBS and recombinant murine Leukemia Inhibitory Factor (LIF) in 5% CO_2 and 37°C.This medium is found to be very useful for culture and derivation of rESC. In this study the whole blastocyst are seeded on the inactivated feeder rather than mechanical isolation of ICM by immunosurgery. The blastocyst stage of embryos those are ready to hatch at the time of collection with bulging of zona pellucida at one point is hatched within 4-6 hours after culture. Embryos those do not show attachment even after of 2-3 days of hatching are discarded and not used for further study. The ICM is allowed to grow on feeder cells for 12-15 days before the first transfer of the growing cells to a new feeder plate. ICM derived outgrowths that are mechanically removed from feeder cells after the perimeter of the outgrowths folded back. The ESC like colonies are mechanically separated from trophoectoderm cells and divided into small clumps by needle, then treated in a drop exposure to 0.05% trpsin-versine solution for 1 minute at room temperature. To terminate digestion, the culture is rinsed once in PBS, resuspended in fresh culture medium, and mechanically disaggregated into small clumps. The small ICM cell clumps are seeded on fresh BFF and the ESC- like colonies are seen several days later. The initial outgrowth of the ICM is often contained heterogeneous cell types. After growing approximately for 6-8 days the colonies are again lifted and passaged further for more separation of cells followed by treatment with 0.05% trypsin-versine solution for few minutes and then propagated in clumps of approximately 500 or more cells on fresh BFF. Embryonic stem cells are expressed high levels of alkaline phosphatase (AP) activity as evidenced by its characteristic pink coloration after staining. Expression of pluripotent markers in cultured embryonic cells is observed by alkaline phosphatase is further confirmed by Oct-4 in few cases by immuno-cytochemistry as evidenced by its green fluorescence. Colonies those shows positive expression are only used for implantation study in segmental bone defect in rabbit model.

The combination of xylazine and ketamine anaesthesia is provided safe and satisfactory anaesthesia for collection of embryos and during the implantation in rabbits and in none of the animals complications due to anaesthesia are observed. The hydroxyapatite -tri calcium phosphate granules are used in the form of granules and are secured at the defect site by suturing surrounding soft tissues. The process of transplantation of embryonic stem cells and growth factors at the site of osteotomy is carried out easily without any complication. Suturing of muscles, soft tissues and skin separately is helped to secure the implants in position and prevented their migration in all animals. External splint application to the respective forelimb immediately after implant application is found very useful to prevent the chances of complete fracture occurrence at the defect site.

Clinically, all the animals of different groups behaved identically, surgical wounds are healed by first intention. All the animals of six groups show signs of lameness in the immediate postoperative period. However, there is no visible difference in lameness between different groups. Weight bearing is gradually improved as signs of inflammation subsided within 8-10 days.

Radiographic observations

The radiographic evaluation is done based on mediolateral view as there is overlapping of the radius by ulna in craniocaudal view. In control group (A), on day 30, a fibrous density appearance is seen near the defect margins and there is no indication of the filling of the defect with newly formed tissue. On day 40, radiological observations are more or less the same except that the newly formed osseous tissue at cut ends is more organized and the fractured ends became more smooth and round. In group B, on day 20, HA-TCP bioceramic granules is appeared relatively more compact with signs of osteogenesis from the periphery. The periosteal reaction is seen adjacent to the cut ends of radius. On day 40, the bone defect is partially filled with newly forming bone; however, the implant is still present. There are indications of slowing down of healing process as the edges appeared relatively smooth and newly formed bone is organized. In group C, on day 10 and 20, the defect site shows increased radiographic density in all animals of this group. The cut ends of the bone are looked hazy and irregular with signs of new bone formation on either ends. On day 30, a radiolucent line is present in the middle of the defect showing incomplete bridging of the gap. On day 40, radiographs show that there are further consolidation of new bone formation and signs of union between the implant and host bone is visible at the proximal end of segmental defect. The implant is looking more compact at this stage indicative of progression of good healing process. In group D, on day 30, there is further increase in new bone formation at the defect site. On day 40, all the animals show signs of increased new bone formation and periosteal reaction at defect site as compared to day 30; however, still there are radiolucent lines visible in between the implant. In group E, on day 20, the signs of new bone formation from both cut ends of radius and radiodensity are increased at the defect site reducing the gap. On day 30, the defect site is completely healed and fused with the adjacent host bone in 4 animals. In remaining animals, new bone growth is seen from bone ends and only a small radiolucent line is visible between the implant and cut end of bone at distal fragment. On day 40, the defect site is appeared more radiodense with complete union between the implant and bone at proximal end of defect. In group F, on day 10, periosteal reaction is started. On day 20, there is increased radiodensity on the defect site, which shows signs of new bone formation. Cartilaginous density is observed at the defect margins on day 30. On day 40 the whole defect shows cartilaginous density whereas the defect margins show bony density and bridging the defect ends.

Histological observations

Histological sections at bone defect site of different groups on day 40 are recorded. In control animals (A), majority of the defect area is occupied by fibrous tissue. However, there is no continuity between fibrous tissue from the proximal and distal fragments. In group B, the defect site shows merging of osteoid bone ingrowths in area adjacent to the fibrous connective tissue with tendency to form Haversian systems and also cavitations lined by many osteoblasts. There are signs of resorption of implanted material. In group C, the histological picture at the defect site shows only partial degradation and absorption of HA-TCP particles. There is no infiltration of any inflammatory cells. However, the connective tissue below the periosteum and underneath the implanted construct mass is moderately thick, having many fibroblasts and osteoblasts with tendency to form Haversian systems and also remodeling with cavitations which are generally lined with osteoblast and also appearance of marrow elements in some of the cavities. The bone defect is almost repaired with newly formed bone. In group D, thick periosteal connective tissue covering over the defect site which is seen invading in and around the implanted bioceramic, which is entrapped within the interlacing osteoid trabeculae. There is evidence of hypertrophied chondrocytes indicating the bone formation through endochondral ossification. The trabecular structures of the bone are lined by many osteoblast cells. In group E, thick band of fibrous connective tissue is seen invading the implanted material from all sides and the interface of the implant-host bone shows intense osteoblastic activity forming woven bony structures having many osteoblasts and few osteoclasts. The new bone formation is found to be comparatively better than groups B and C. In group F, mild to moderate amount of implanted material is getting embedded into mature bony tissue having developed Haversian system. The osteoid tissue is more prominent forming woven bone pattern and the stroma consisted of large number of osteoblasts and osteocytes. There is complete filling of the defect area by new bone growth. The interlacing bony trabeculae are seen covering grafted material at the defect site. The margins of the trabecular bone are lined by osteoblasts and osteoclasts cells.

Scanning Electron Microscopic (SEM) study

SEM analyses at bone defect site of different groups on day 40 are recorded. In group A, the gap is filled by newly proliferated tissue which is a mixture of cartilaginous and fibrous tissues. The fibro cartilage is present at the centre of the defect. Adjacent periosteal surface of the ulna is also attached with healing site through newly proliferated tissues. However, it is only fibroblast that invaded the defect. In group B, HA-TCP particles are seen projecting over the surface. These particles are seen surrounded by newly formed bone matrix suggesting that bioceramic provided base for new bone formation, however, it is failed to incorporate with newly formed bones. In group C, the healing process of new bone formation is relatively faster as compared to group B. The ceramic particles are seen fused with newly formed bone matrix suggesting their incorporation with newly formed osseous tissue. Unorganized osseous tissue is advanced from the cut edges into the implant material. The area of the implanted site is almost completely occupied by the bone matrix. The extracellular matrix is well organized at many places indicating maturity of the osseous tissue. In group D, the defect site reveals some irregular area in the centre and at the host implant junction there is presence of compact bone suggesting advanced stage of healing. In group E, the SEM picture depicts compact bone formation at the host and implant junction towards the periosteal surface of the bones. Further magnification of the implanted site shows well organized trabecular bone embedded in the implanted material which is surrounded by compact bone at places. In group F, scanning micrograph of healing site shows some irregular areas in the centre of the defect and at the junction of the bioceramic construct and the cut edges, there is presence of compact bone suggesting advance stage of healing.

In conclusion, adding of allogenous rESC on bioscaffold HA-TCP can hasten the osteoconductive properties of bioceramic and can be alternative to autogenous bone graft in the treatment of delayed and non-union. Addition of growth proteins includes BMP-2, TGF-ß and IGF-1 to ESC seeded HA-TCP bioceramic construct could accelerate bone regeneration in a segmental bone defect model controlled study.

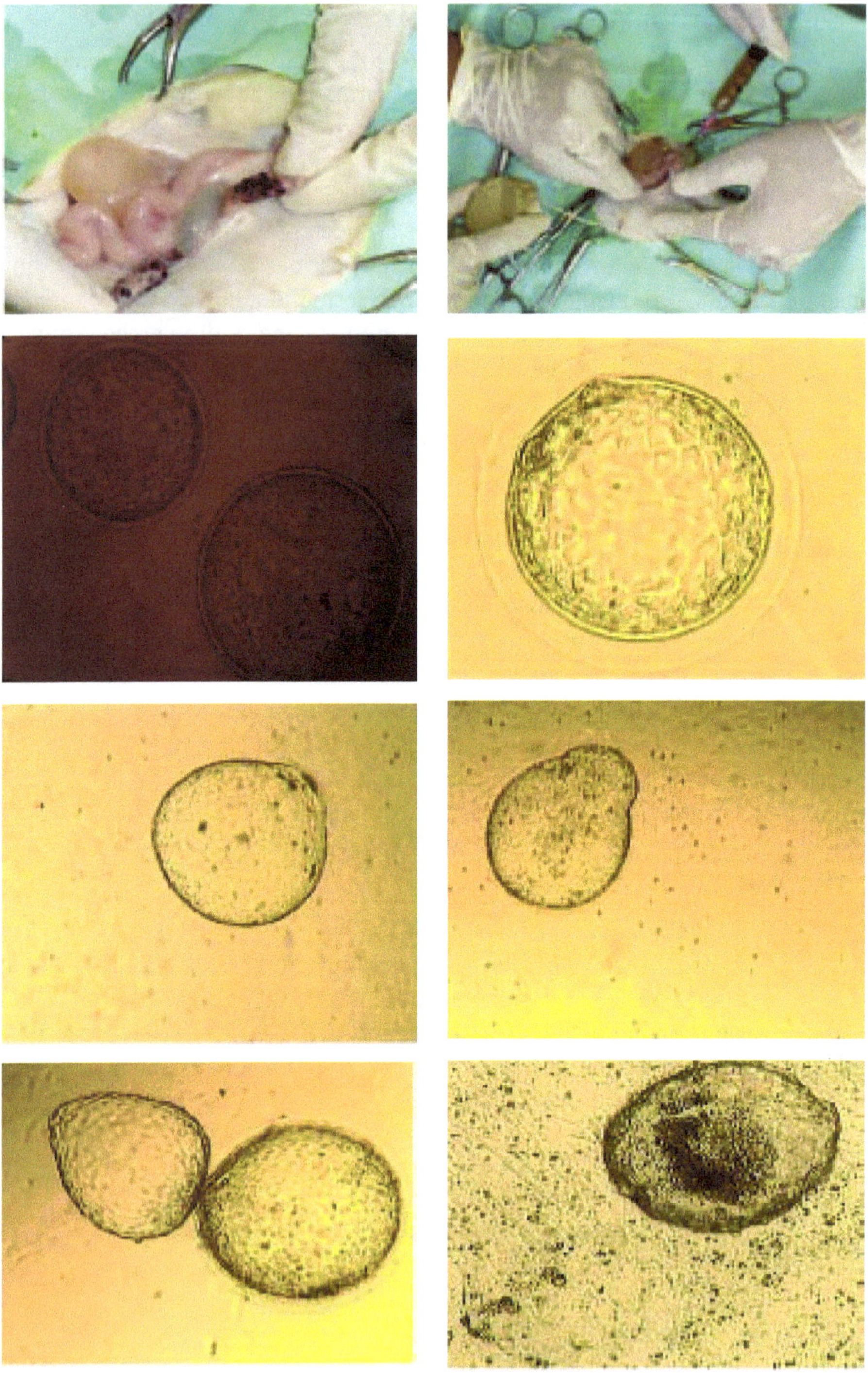

Procedure for embryo collection

Procedure for embryo collection

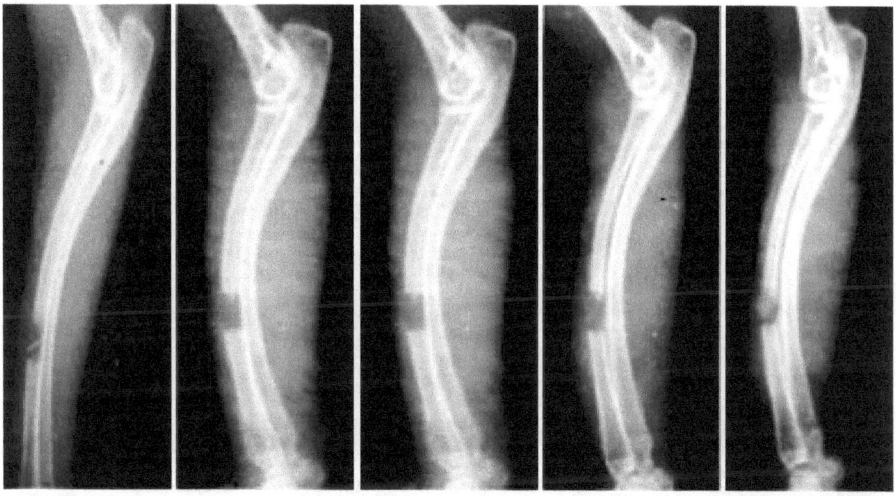

Day 0 10 20 30 40

Sequential radiographs of gr A

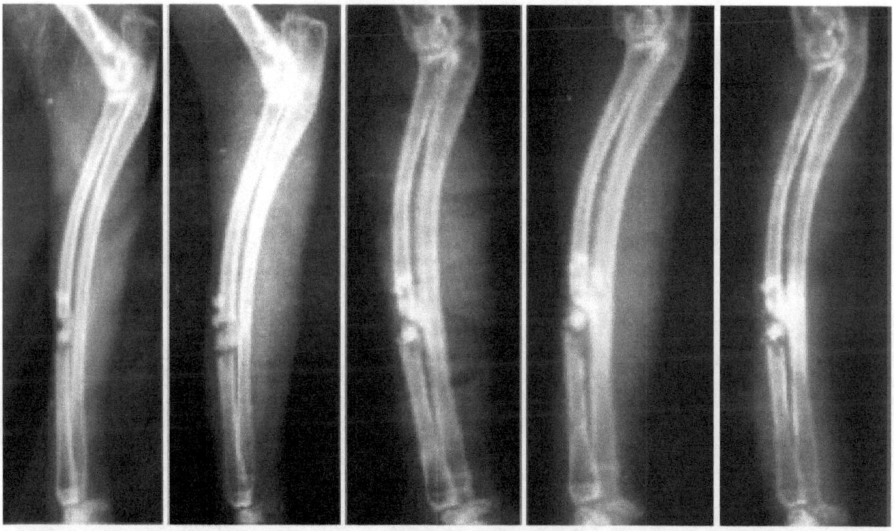

Day 0 10 20 30 40

Sequential radiographs of gr B

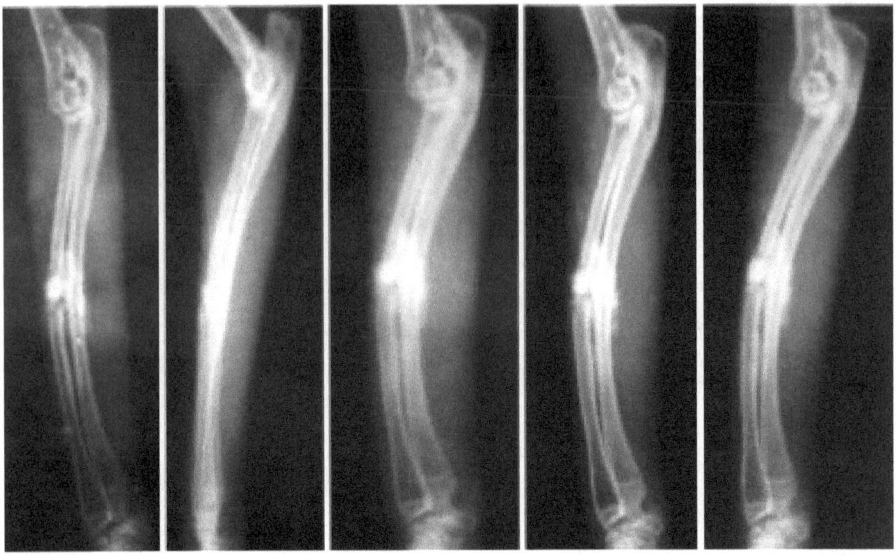

Day 0 10 20 30 40

Sequential radiographs of gr C

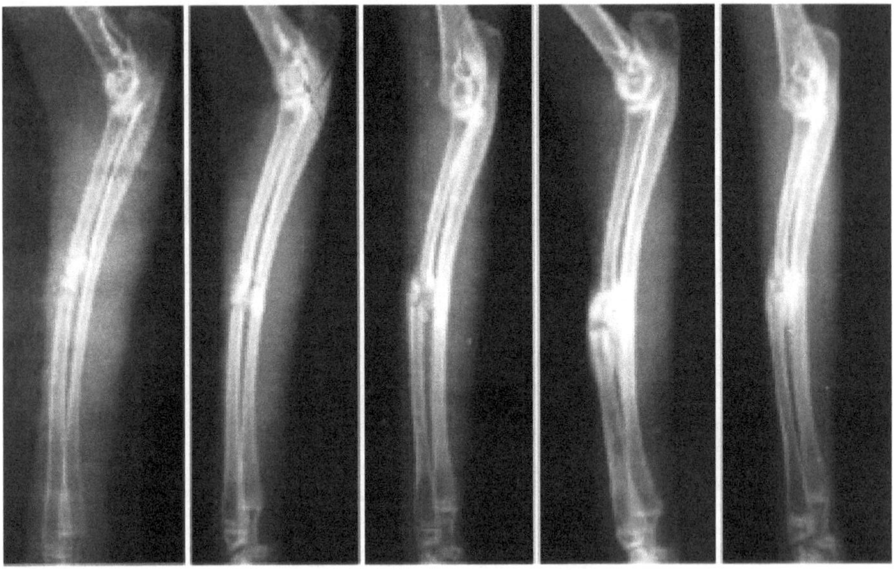

Day 0 10 20 30 40

Sequential radiographs of gr D

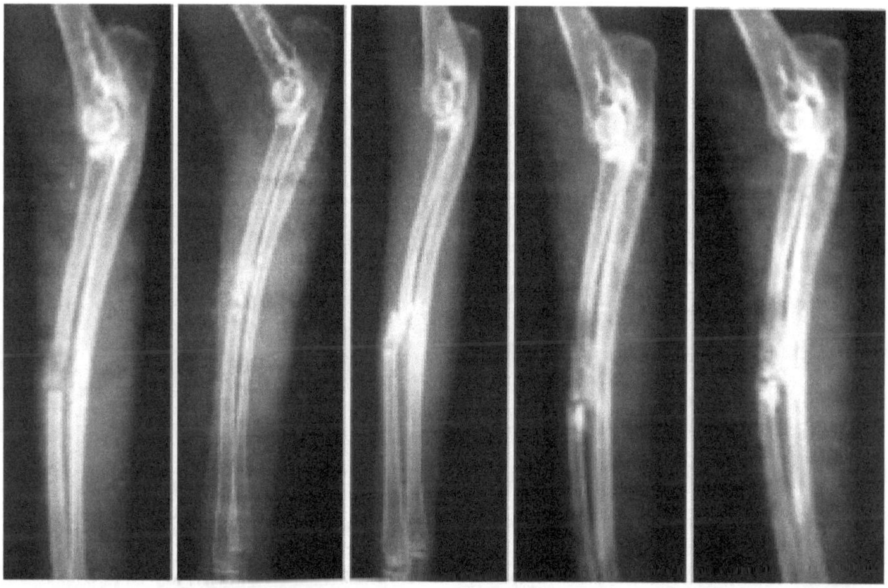

Day 0 10 20 30 40

Sequential radiographs of gr E

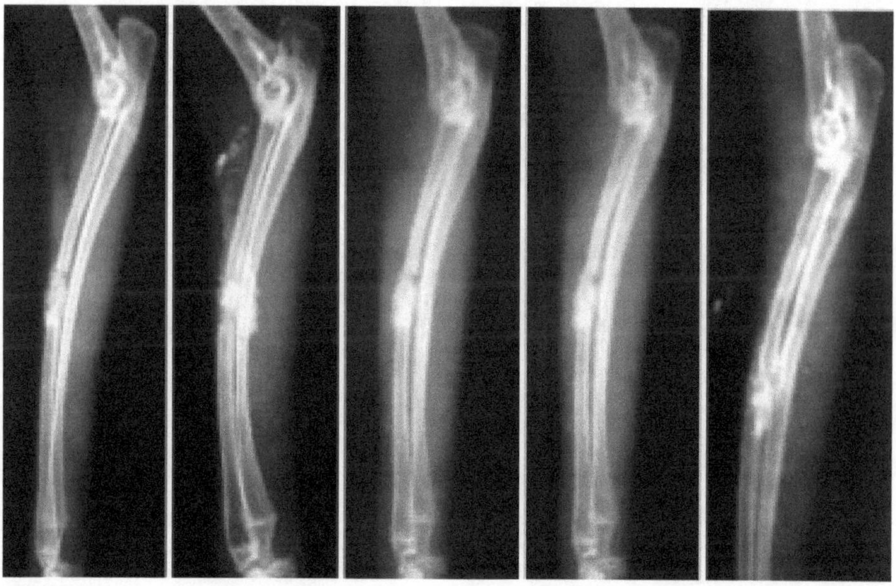

Day 0 10 20 30 40

Sequential radiographs of gr F

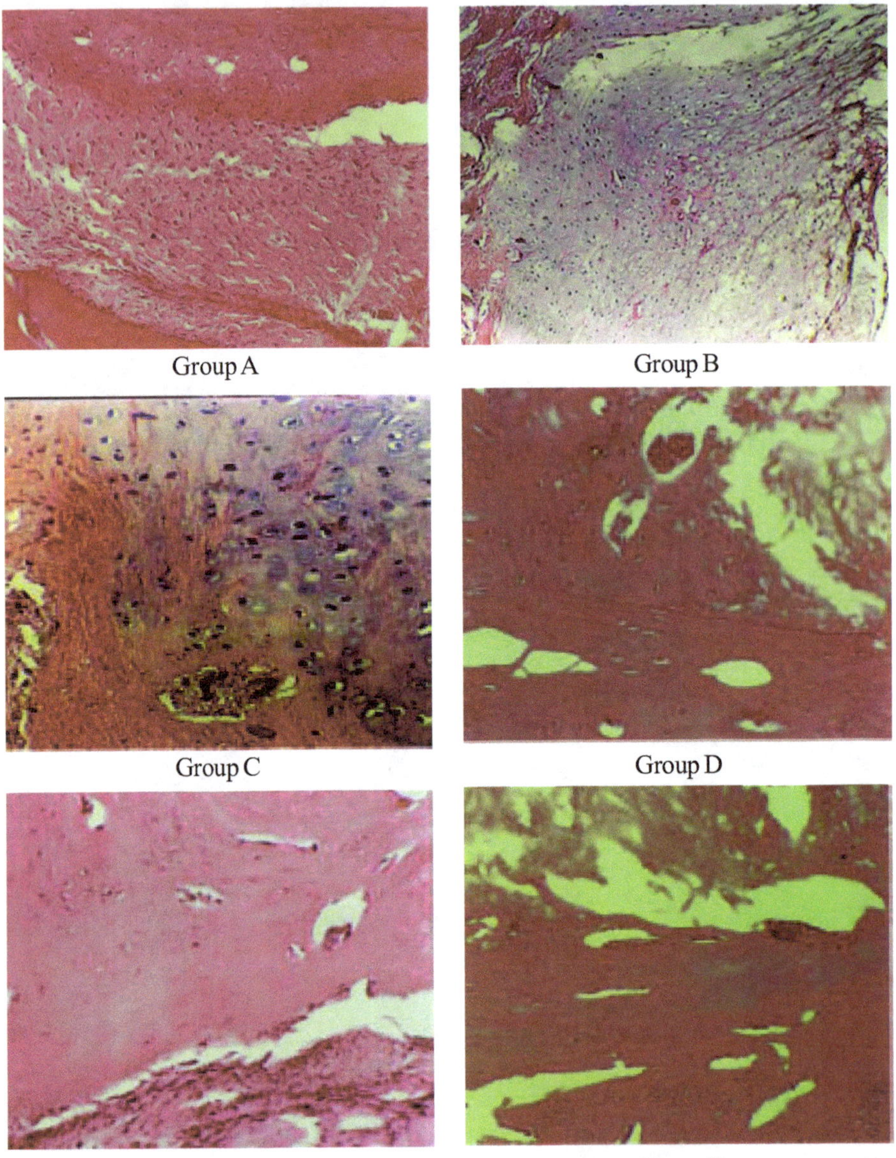

Histological observations of different groups

14

Protocol for Bone-marrow Derived MSC Isolation from Rat

1. Collect the femur and tibia and clean them very well from blood, tendons, muscle, skin and other tissues (using scalpel)
2. Cut off epi-and metaphysis from the long bones with electric/manual bone saw
3. Transfer the open bones to a falcon tubes containing cell culture medium/ DPBS without FBS but containing 1% PS (Penicillin-streptomycin)
4. Transfer the bones to a Petri dish containing 5 ml medium without serum (FBS) and without antibiotic (40-50 mm Petri dish)
5. Remove the pteri dish to the laminar cabinet
6. Collect the bone marrow by flushing out to a 50 ml falcon tube (use syringes and needles to flush out the bone marrow; flush out the bone marrow with complete (10% FBS, 1% PS, 90% DMEM-LG) culture medium
7. Centrifugation: 300rpm, 8 min (in the meanwhile prepare 5 ml of Ficoll into a 15ml falcon tube)
8. Aspire the medium
9. Resuspend the cell pellet with complete medium using the same volume of Ficoll, thus, 5 ml of medium
10. Carefully add the cell suspension into the Ficoll containing falcon tubes.

    (Note: add the cell suspension very carefully through the wall of the falcon tubes)

    Allow 2 phases to form-media, Interface with stem cell, Ficoll and at bottom Blood clot
11. Centrifugation: 2500 rpm, 30 min

12. Collect the interface containing the stem cells using 1ml micropipette
13. Add complete culture medium (9ml); Mix well; Centrifugation: 1500 rpm, 15 minutes
14. Resuspend the cell pallet with complete culture medium (90 ml DMEM-LG; 10 ml FBS, 1 ml PS)
15. Place the cells into a T-75 flask with fresh complete culture medium (P0)-kept in CO_2 incubator at 5% CO_2, 21% O_2 at 37^{0}C.
16. Allow the MSC to be adhere with plastic wall of the flask for 4-5 days

    -Do not change the media during these days; instead add fresh medium-if necessary.

15

Protocol for Fat Derived MSC Isolation from Rat

1. Collect fat tissues from euthanized animals into a Falcon tube containing DPBS + 1% PS (for transferring lab to lab)
2. Wash 3 times with DPBS + 1% PS
3. Inside a laminar cabinet, transfer the fat to a Petridis (use an sterile spatula to collect the fat)
4. Cut the fat into small (mm) pieces using scalpel and forceps or scissors
5. Transfer the fat into a Falcon tube (eg into a 50 ml Falcon tube you can add upto 10 ml fat tissues)
6. Wash the fat by adding approx 40 ml DPBS; Centrifugation: 430g, 10 min (without break)
7. Transfer the fat into a fresh 50 ml Falcon tube (with the help of sterile spatula); Repeat steps 5 to 7 for 2-3 times
8. Add equal volume of collagen type II solution for fat (Aliquots: -20°C : 20mg/ml; eg. 100 mg Col II in 5ml in 5 ml HBSS, sterile filtration in 20μm blue filter and store in -20°C); Concentration for digestion: approx 0.4 mg/ml; eg for 12 ml fat tissues add 110 μl Col II stock solution)
9. Incubate the mixtures at 37°C using a water bath for 30 min
10. Add pre-warm complete culture medium (10% FBS, 1% PS, 90% DMEM-LG) up to 50 ml to stop the collageneage
11. Mix carefully; Centrifugation: 600g for 10 min
12. Remove the upper layer of fat to a Petridis with the forceps or spatula
13. Aspire the media
14. Resuspend the pellet with complete culture media (eg 12 ml)
15. Filtrate the suspension through a cell strainer (BD, blue, 40μm into a fresh 50 ml Falcon tube

16. Add fresh complete culture media (eg 15 ml) and transfer the cell suspension to a culture flask (T-75)
17. To remove the non-adherent cells, like RBC, change the culture media the first day after isolation (P0)
18. Remove the culture media from T-75 flask
19. Wash with DPBS X 3 times (DPBS-1X); Remove DPBS completely
20. Add 5 ml Aqutus for cell lifting; Kept flask in CO_2 incubator for 5 min
21. Add 5 ml fresh media for de-Aqutus effect for 5 min
22. Collect all the lifting cell into a 50 ml Falcon tube
23. Centrifuge the collected cell + media + Aqutus for 1100 rpm for 8 min
24. Aspire the media, Discard
25. Wash the cell pallet with DPBS; Remove DPBS completely
26. Add Media (3ml), gently mix with cell pellet
27. Cell Count, Divide into three T-75 flak (1ml with 5 ml complete media), Kept in CO_2 incubator for P1

16

Protocol for Bone Marrow Derived MSC Isolation from Rabbit, Dog, Goat, Sheep and Pig

1. Collect the bone marrow from iliac crest of rabbit, dog, goat and sheep; sternum of pigs by 16-18 G bone marrow biopsy needle under sedation/ anesthesia and maintain strict asepsis protocol
2. To aspirate bone marrow, negative pressure should create in the syringe by pulling back the plunger. Syringe should be first flushed with heparin before bone marrow collection
3. Collect approximately 2.5-5 ml of bone marrow from each animal
4. Mix the bone marrow sample with equal volume of low DMEM having 10% FBS and 1 ml of PS and then layer on 5 ml of histopaque/Ficol-Paque Plus in a falcon tube
5. Centrifuge at 3000 rpm for 30 min
6. Collect stem cells from the interface with the help of a micropipette
7. Cells wash thrice with DPBS
8. Centrifuged at 2000 rpm for 5 min
9. Cells resuspend in complete growth medium (10% FBS, 1% PS, 90% DMEM-LG) in T-25/75 flask and maintain at 37°C in a humidified atmosphere of 5% CO_2 and 95% air in a CO_2 incubator
10. After 3-5 days of primary culture, non-adherent cells should be removed by completely changing the medium
11. The medium should be change on every 3rd days thereafter.
12. The spindle shape, fibroblast like MSC grows as symmetrical colonies within 14-18 days
13. Upon reaching 80% confluence, the cells should passage into new culture flasks

17

Protocol for Mesenchymal Stem cell Passaging

1. Remove the growth media
2. Wash 2 times with warm PBS (w/o Ca and Mg)
3. Add 5ml of trypsin /EDTA 0.35 % (Invitrogen), place at 37^{0}C in a CO_2 incubator for 4-5 min
4. Wait until cells are detached/lifted and make sure by examining on microscope
5. Add equal volume (5ml-1:1) of growth medium as appropriate and mix with 5 strokes
6. Transfer into 15 ml centrifuge tube
7. Centrifuge at room temperature for 4 min in 980 rpm
8. Remove supernatant complete but carefully without touching the cell aliquot
9. Re-suspend in 10ml DPBS (with Ca and Mg)-5 strokes
10. Immediately after mixing transfer 100µl of cell suspension into Casy vial, containing 10ml Casyton
11. Proceed to Casy machine and arrange the spectrum (0-30 µm), cursors left at 8.25 µm and right at 30 µm. (CL:08.25 µm, CR:30.00 µm)
12. Take an aliquot of 500000 cells and transfer into new 50ml tube
13. Centrifuge at above
14. Remove supernatant completely without touching the cell palate
15. Re-suspend the pellet in 50 ml of complete medium, mix well by turning the tube
16. Place 2 ml of cell suspension /well into a 24-wells, mix well and place at 37^{0}C in a CO_2 incubator (5% CO_2, 21 % O_2)

17. In absence of Casy machine, cells may be count by Neubar's counting chamber method and place at an average 2.2 x 10^5 cells/cm in one T-25 flask and then maintain in a CO_2 incubator.

References & Further Reading

Agrawal S, Pittenger MF. (2005) Human mesenchymal stem cells modulate allogeneic immune cell responses. Blood, 105:1815-22.

Arinzeh, T. L. (2005) Mesenchymal Stem Cells for Bone Repair: Preclinical Studies and Potential Orthopedic Applications. Foot and Ankle Clinics of North America., 10: 651-665.

Arinzeh, T. L., Peter, S. J., Archambault, M. P., Van Den bos, C., Gordon, S., Kraus. K., Smith, A. and Kadiyala, S. (2003) Allogeneic Mesenchymal Stem Cells Regenerate Bone in a Critical-Sized Canine Segmental Defect. J. Bone. Joint. Surg. Am., 85A: 1927.

Arinzeh, T. L., Tranb, T., Mcalaryb, J. and Daculsic, G. (2005) A comparative study of biphasic calcium phosphate ceramics for human mesenchymal stem-cell induced bone formation. Biomaterials, 26: 3631–3638.

Atiyeh, B.S., Gunn, S.W. and Hayek, S.N. (2005) State of the art in burn treatment. World Journal of Surgery 29: 131-148.

Awad HA, Butler DL, *et al.* (1999) Autologous mesenchymal stem cell-mediated repair of tendon. Tissue Eng., 5:267-77.

Badylak, S. F. (1993) Small intestinal submucosa (SIS): a biomaterial conducive to smart tissue remodeling. In: E. BELL (eds): Tissue Engineering: Current Perspectives, Birkenhäuser, Boston. pp 179-189.

Badylak, S. F., Coffey, A. C., Lantz, G. C., Tacker, W. A. and Geddes L. A. (1994) Comparison of the resistance to infection of intestinal submucosa arterial autografts versus polytetrafluoroethylene arterial prostheses in a dog model. J. Vasc. Surg. 19: 465-472.

Badylak, S., Liang, A., Record, R., Tullius, R. and Hodde, J. (1999) Endothelial cell adherence to small intestinal submucosa: An acellular bioscaffold. Biomaterials, 20: 2257–2263.

Barrilleaux, B., Phinney, D. G., Prockop, D. J., and O'Connor, K. C. (2006) Review: Ex vivo engineering of living tissues with adult stem cells. Tissue Eng., 12: 3007–3019.

Barry, F. P. and Murphy, J. M. (2004) Mesenchymal stem cells: Clinical applications and biological characterization. Int. J. Biochem Cell Biol., 36:568–584.

Baur TW, Smith ST. (2002) Bioactive materials in orthopedics surgery: overview and regulatory considerations. Clin Orthop Rev., 395:11-22.

Beyer, N. N. and da Silva Meirelles, L. (2006) Mesenchymal stem cells: Isolation, in vitro expansion and characterization. Hand Exp Pharmacol., pp: 249–282.

Bhadane, B. and Maiti, S.K. (2011) Role of embryonic stem cells for osteogenesis in the repair of bone defects in rabbit model. 35th Annual Conference of ISVS (Kolkata) Abstract no-OS-OP-11, P-177.

Bhadane, B, Maiti S K, Mohan Divya, Bag S and Kumar N (2018) Role of embryonic stem cell-hydroxyapatite construct with growth proteins for osteogenesis in the repair if bone defects in rabbit model. Journal of Stem Cell Research & Therapeutics, 4(4):67-80.

Bianco, P. and Gehron, R. P. (2000) Marrow stromal stem cells. J. Clin. Invest. 105: 1663–1668

Bjelakovic G, Nagorni A, Bjelokovic M, Stamenkovic I, Arsic R, Katic V. (2005) Apoptosis: programmed cell death and its clinical implications. Medicine and Biology 12: 6 – 11.

Bobis S, Jarocha D and Majka M (2006) Mesenchymal stem cells: characteristics and clinical applications. Folia Histochemica Et Cytobiologica, 44: 215-230.

Bolander, M. E. and Balian, G. (1986) The use of demineralized bone matrix in the repair of segmental defects augmentation with extracted matrix proteins and comparison with autologous grafts. J. Bone Joint Surg., 68-A: 1264-1274.

Bongso A and Lee EH (2010) Stem cells: Their definition, classification and sources (Chapter 1). In, Stem Cells from Bench to Beside, 2nd Edition, World Scientific Publishing Co Pvt Ltd, New Jersey, Chennai.

Bourin P, Gadelorge M, Peyrafitte JA, Cappellesso S F, Gomez M, Rage C and Sensebe L (2008) Mesenchymal Progenitor Cells: Tissue Origin, Isolation and Culture. Transfus Med Hemother, 35: 160-67.

Brighton CT, Hunt RM (1991) Early histological and ultrastructural changes in medullary fracture callus. The Journal of Bone and Joint Surgery. 73: 832–47.

Brown, B., Lindberg, K., Reing, J., Stolz, D.B. and Badylak, S.F. (2006) The basement membrane component of biologic scaffolds derived from extracellular matrix. Tissue engineering 12: 519-526.

Bruder SP, Jaiswal N, Kadiyala S, *et al.* (1998) Mesenchymal stem cells in osteobiology and applied bone regeneration. Clin Orthop Relat Res, 355 Suppl: S247-256.

Bruder, S. P., Kraus, K. H., Goldberg, V. M. and Kadiyala, S. (1998) The effect of implants loaded with autologous mesenchymal stem cells on the healing of canine segmental bone defects. J. Bone Joint Surg. Am., 80: 985–996.

Calloni R, Viegas GS, Turck P, Bonatto D and Henriques JAP (2014) Mesenchymal stromal cells from unconventional model organisms. Cytotherapy, 16:3.

Caplan A I (1991) Mesenchymal stem cells. J Orthop Res, 9: 641–50.

Caplan AI (2007) Adult mesenchymal stem cells for tissue engineering versus regenerative medicine. J Cell Physiol 213: 341-347.

Caplan AI, (2006) Mesenchymal stem cells. In: Essential of stem cell biology. Edited by Lanza R, Gearhart J, Hogan B, Melton D, Pedersen R, Thomson J, Thomas ED and West M Elsevier Co Ltd London, pp: 205-210.

Chen J, Li Y, Wang L, Zhang Z, Lu D, Lu M, Chopp M. (2001) Therapeutic benefit of intravenous administration of bone marrow stromal cells after cerebral ischemia in rats. Stroke, 32: 1005-1011.

Chen J, Zhang ZG, Li Y, Wang L, Xu YX, Gautam SC, Lu M, Zhu Z, Chopp M. (2003) Intravenous administration of human bone marrow stromal cells induces angiogenesis in the ischemic boundary zone after stroke in rats. Circ Res. 92:692-9.

Chen, M.K. and Badylak, S.F. (2001) Small bowel tissue engineering using small intestinal submucosa as a scaffold. Journal of Surgical Research 99: 352-358.

Clark RAF and MD Denver (1985) Cutaneous tissue repair: Basic biologic considerations. J Amer Acad Dermatol, 13: 701-725.

Clarke, K. M., Lantz, G. C., Salisbury, S. K., Badylak, S. F., Hiles, M. C. and Voytik, S.L. (1996) Intestine submucosa and polypropylene mesh for abdominal wall repair in dogs. J. Surg. Res. 60: 107-114.

Conti B, P Giunchedi, I Genta and U Conte (2000) The preparation and in vivo evaluation of the wound healing properties of chitosan microspheres. STP Pharm Sci, 10: 101-104.

Cowan CM, Shi YY, Aalami OO, *et al.* (2004) Adipose-derived adult stromal cells heal critical-size mouse calvarial defects. Nat Biotechnol, 22:560-7.

Crapo, P.M., Gilbert, T.W. and Badylak, S.F. (2011) An overview of tissue and whole organ decellularization processes. Biomaterials 32: 3233-3243.

-Daculsi G, Passuti N, Martin S, Deudon C, Legeros RZ, Raher S. (1990) Macroporous calcium phosphate ceramic for long bone surgery in humans and dogs. Clinical and histological study. J Biomed Mater Res., 24:379-96.

Dai, K. R., Xu, X. L., Tang, T. T., Zhu, Z. A., Yu, C. F. and Lou, J. R. (2005) Repairing of goat Tibial Bone Defects with BMP-2 Gene-Modified Tissue-Engineered Bone. Calcif. Tissue Int., 77: 55–61.

Davies, J.E. (2007) Bone bonding at natural and biomaterial surfaces. Biomaterials, 28: 5058-5067.

Deans RJ, Moseley AB (2000) Mesenchymal stem cells: biology and potential clinical uses. Exp Hematol 28(8): 875-884.

De-Kolk IJ, Drapeau SJ, Young R and Cooper LF (2005) Evaluation of mesenchymal stem cells following implantation in alveolar sockets: a canine safety study. Int J Oral Maxillofac Implants, 20: 511-518.

De-Kolk IJ, Peter SJ, Archambault M *et al*., (2003) Investigation of allogenic mesenchymal stem cell- based alveolar bone formation: preliminary findings. Clin Oral Impl. Res., 14: 481-489.

Divya Mohan (2018) Evaluation of mesenchymal stem cells with conditioned media and m-EGF for regeneration of liver tissue after partial hepatectomy in rats. Ph D Thesis submitted to the IVRI Deemed University.

Devescovi V, Leonardi E, Ciapetti G, Cenni E. (2008) Growth factors in bone repair. Chir Organi Mov., 92:161-68.

Dezawa M, Kanno H, Hoshino M, Cho H, Matsumoto N, *et al.* (2004) Specific induction of neuronal cells from bone marrow stromal cells and application for autologous transplantation. J Clin Invest 113: 1701-1710.

Dominici M, Hofmann TJ, Horwitz EM (2001) Bone marrow mesenchymal cells: biological properties and clinical applications. J Biol Regul Homeost Agents 15: 28-37.

Dominici M, Le Blanc K, Mueller I, Slaper-Cortenbach I, Marini F, Krause D, Deans R, Keating A, Prockop DJ and Horwitz E (2006) Minimal criteria for defining multipotent mesenchymal stromal cells. The International Society for Cellular Therapy position statement. Cytotherapy, 8: 315-27.

Duchyene P, Qiu Q (1999) Bioactive ceramics: the effect of surface reactivity on bone formation and bone cell function. Biomaterials 29: 2287-2303.

Ehrbar, M., Zeisberger, S.M., Raeber, G.P., Hubbell, J.A., Schnell, C. and Zisch, A.H. (2008) The role of actively released fibrin-conjugated VEGF for VEGF receptor 2 gene activation and the enhancement of angiogenesis. Biomaterials 29: 1720-1729.

EI Ghannam AR (2004) Advanced bioceramic composite for bone tissue engineering: design principles and structure-bioactivity relationship. J Biomed Mater Res A 69: 490-501.

Eslaminejad MB, Nadri S, Hosseini RH (2007) Expression of Thy 1.2 surface antigen increases significantly during the murine mesenchymal stem cells cultivation period. Dev Growth Differ 49(4): 351-364.

Ettinger, M. (2003) Aging bone and osteoporosis: Strategies for preventing fractures in the elderly. Arch. Intern. Med., 163: 2237– 2246.

Fatkhudinov T Kh, Gol'dshtein DV, Pullin AA etal., (2005) Reparative osteogenesis during transplantation of mesenchymal stem cells. Bulletin of Experimental Biology and Medicine, 140: 96-99.

Fiedler J, Brill C, Blum WF, Brenner RE. (2006) IGF-1 and IGF-2 stimulate directed cell migration of bone marrow derived human mesenchymal progenitor cells. Biochem Biophys Res Comm., 345: 1177-83.

Friedenstein A J, Chailakhyan R K, Latsinik NV, Panasyuk A F and Keiliss-Borok I V (1974) Stromal cells responsible for transferring the microenvironment of the hemopoietic tissues. Cloning in vitro and retransplantation in vivo. Transplantation, 17: 331-40.

Friedenstein A J, Petrakova KV, Kurolesova A I and Frolova G P (1968) Heterotopic of bone marrow. Analysis of precursor cells for osteogenic and hematopoietic tissues. Transplantation, 6: 230-47.

Friedenstein, A. J. (1990) Osteogenic stem cells in bone marrow. In Bone and Mineral Research, J. N. M. Heersche and J.A. Kanis, eds. (Amsterdam: Elsevier), pp. 243–272.

Friedenstein, A.J., Chailakhyan, R.K. and Gerasimov, U.V. (1987) Bone marrow osteogenic stem cells: in vitro cultivation and transplantation in diffusion chambers. Cell Tissue Kinet. 20(3):263-726.

Gajiwala, K. and Gajiwala, A.L. (2004) Evaluation of lyophilised, gamma-irradiated amnion as a biological dressing. Cell and Tissue Banking 5: 73-80.

Ganguly NK and Bhan MK (2007) Guidelines for Stem Cell Research and Therapy. Published by Department of Biotechnology and Indian Council of Medical Research, New Delhi.

Gilbert, T.W., Stewart-Akers, A.M., Simmons-Byrd, A. and Badylak, S.F. (2007) Degradation and remodeling of small intestinal submucosa in canine Achilles tendon repair. The Journal of Bone & Joint Surgery 89: 621-630.

Gilger, B. C. (2007) Diseases and Surgery of the Canine Cornea and Sclera. In: Veterinary Ophthalmology. 4th ed. K. N. Gelatt (ed.). Ames: Blackwell Publishing. 690-752.

Gopinathan A, Sigh K, Sangeetha P and Maiti S K (2018) Evaluation of caprine amniotic membrane and rabbit mesenchymal stem cells for corneal defect repair in rabbits. Indian Journal of Small Ruminants 24 (1): 110-114.

Harris CT and Cooper LF (2004) Comparison of bone graft matrices for human mesenchymal stem cell –directed osteogenesis. J Biomed Mater Res, 68A:747-755.

Hayashi, S., Osawa, T. and Tohyama, K. (2002) Comparative observations on corneas, with special reference to Bowman's layer and Descement's membrane in mammals and amphibians. J Morphol. 254: 247–258.

Haynesworth, S. E., Reuben, D., and Caplan, A. I. (1998) Cell-based tissue engineering therapies: The influence of whole body physiology. Adv. Drug Deliv. Rev., 33: 3–14.

Heersche, J. N., Bellows, C. G and Ishida, Y. (1998) The decrease in bone mass associated with aging and menopause. J. Prosthet. Dent., 79: 14–16.

Hench, L. L. and Polak, J. M., (2002) Third-Generation Biomedical Materials. Science, 295: 1014

Herndon, D.N. and Parks, D.H. (1986) Comparison of serial debridement and autografting and early massive excision with cadaver skin overlay in the treatment of large burns in children. Journal of Trauma and Acute Care Surgery 26: 149-152.

Hutmacher DW and Sugunan SLC (2010) Bone repair and Adult Stem Cells (Chapter 21). In, Stem Cells from Bench to Beside, 2nd Edition, World Scientific Publishing Co Pvt Ltd, New Jersey, Chennai, P-442.

Http//www. Mesenchymal Stem cell Wikipedia

Ishihara M, K Nakanishi, K Ono, M Sato, M Kikuchi and Y Saito (2002) Photo cross linkable chitosan as a dressing for wound occlusion and accelerator in healing process. Biomaterials, 23: 833-40.

Jaiswal N, Haynesworth S E, Caplan A I, and Bruder S P (1997) Osteogenic differentiation of purified, culture-expanded human mesenchymal stem cell in vitro. J Cell Biochem, 64: 295-312.

Jeong JH, Ki YW, Kim JY, Jan SH, Kim SH, Chang Y. (2005) Adipose Tissue Derived MSC Enhances Motor Function in Rats with Cerebral Infarction. IFATS, Oral Presentation

Jia L, Young MF, Powell J, Yang L, Ho NC, *et al.* (2002) Gene expression profile of human bone marrow stromal cells: high-throughput expressed sequence tag sequencing analysis. Genomics 79: 7-17.

Jiang, X., Cui, P. and Chen, W. (2002) Study on the directed inducing process of cartilage cells differentiated from human marrow Mesenchymal stem cells. Zhonghua Er Bi Yan Hou Ke Za Zhi 37: 137–139.

Jori F P, Napolitano M A and Melone M A (2005) Molecular pathways involved in neural in vitro differentiation of marrow stromal stem cells. J Cell Biochem, 94: 645–655.

Joseph, M. L., Emre, T. and Mathias P. G. B (1999) Biosynthetic bone grafting. Clin. Orthop., 36: 107.

Kadiyala, S., Young, R.G., Thiede, M.A. and Bruder, S.P. (1997) Culture expanded canine mesenchymal stem cells possess osteochondrogenic potential in vivo and in vitro. Cell Tran., 6: 125–1349-

Kasten P, Vogel J, Luginbuhl R, Niemeyer P, Tonak M, Lorenz H. (2005) Ectopic bone formation associated with mesenchymal stem cells in a resorbable calcium deficient hydroxyapatite carrier. Biomaterials, 26: 5879-89.

Kim H-J, Park J-B, Lee J-K, Park E-Y, Park E-A, Riew K Daniel and Rhee S-K (2008) Transplanted xenoxenic bone marrow stem cells survive and generate new bone formation in the posterolateral lumber spine of non-immunosuppressed rabbits. Eur Spine J, 17: 1515-21.

Kon, E., Muraglia, A., Corsi, A., Bianco, P., Marcacci, M., Martin, I., Boyde, A., Ruspantini, I., Chistolini, P., Rocca, M., Giardino, R., Cancedda, R. and Quarto, R. (2000) Autologous bone marrow stromal cells loaded onto porous hydroxyapatite ceramic accelerate bone repair in critical-size defects of sheep long bones. J. Biomed. Mater. Res., 49:328–337.

Kortesidis A, Zannettino A, Isenmann S, Shi S, Lapidot T, Gronthos S. (2005) Stromal-derived factor-1 promotes the growth, survival, and development of human bone marrow stromal stem cells. Blood, 105:3793-801.

Kraus K H and Kirker-Head C (2006) Mesenchymal stem cells and bone regeneration-Invited Review. Vet Surg, 35: 232-242.

Kumar, A., Maiti, S. K., Ninu AR, Balwada, A. K., Mathew, D. D. and Kumar, N. (2014) The Effects of Topical Mesenchymal Stem Cell Therapy in Full Thickness Skin Wound Healing in a Rat Model. Trends Biomater. Artif. Organs. 28: 65-73.

Langer R and Vacanti J P (1993) Tissue engineering. Science, 260: 920-26.

Lapi S, Nocchi F, Lamanna R, Passeri S, Iorio M, Paolicchi A, Urciuoli P, Coli A, Abramo F, Miragliotta V, Giannessi E, Stornelli M R, Vanacore R, Stampacchia G, Pisani G, Borghetti L and Scatena F (2008) Different media and supplements modulate the clonogenic and expansionproperties of rabbit bone marrow mesenchymal stem cells. BMC Res Note, 1: 53.

Lendeckel S, Jodicke A, Christophis P, *et al.* (2004) Autologous stem cells (adipose) and fibrin glue used to treat widespread traumatic calvarial defects: case report. J Craniomax Surg 32:370-373.

Li Ye, Chen SK, Li L, Qin L, Wang XL, Lai YX. (2015) Bone defect animal models for testing efficacy of bone substitute biomaterials. J Orthop Translatiom 3: 95-104.

Linkhart TA, Mohan S, Baylink DJ. (1996) Growth factors for bone growth and repair: IGF, TGF-beta and BMP. Bone 19 (1 Suppl): 1S-12S.

-Liu, C. Z., and Czernuszka, J. T. (2007) On the process capability of the solid free-form fabrication: A case study of scaffold moulds for tissue engineering Mater. Sci. Technol., 23: 379–392.

Lotfy A, Salama M, Zahran F, Jones E, Badawy A, *et al.* (2014) Characterization of mesenchymal stem cells derived from rat bone marrow and adipose tissue: a comparative study. Int J Stem Cells 7: 135-142.

Lutolf MP, Hubbell JA (2005) Synthetic biomaterials as instructive extracellular microenvironments for morphogenesis in tissue engineering. Nat Biotechnol 23: 47-55.

Ma'rquez SP, MartinezVS, AmbroseWM, Wang J, Gantxegui NG, Schein O, and Elisseeff J (2009) Decellularization of bovinecorneas for tissue engineering. Acta Biomaterialia 5: 1839-1847.

Maiti S K (2017) Tissue engineered construct of mesenchymal stem cells seeded with different biomaterials for skin wound repair, Final Research Report submitted to Indian Veterinary Research Institute, Izatnagar as Principal Investigator.

Maiti S K, Ferguson James G, Ionita Jean-Claude (2008) Mesenchymal stem cell construct for osteogenesis in swine XVth Annual Conference of Indian Association for the Advancement of Veterinary Research, Kolkata, Compendium, p-200.

Maiti S K, Ninu A R, Sangeetha P, Mathew D D, Tamilmahan P, Kritaniya D, Kumar N and Hescheler J (2016) Mesenchymal stem cells-seeded bioceramic construct for bone regeneration in large critical-size bone defect in rabbit. Journal of Stem Cells & Regenerative Medicine, 12; 87-99.

Maiti S K, Shiva Kumar MU, Srivastava L, Kumar N, Ninu AR. (2012) Isolation, proliferation and morphological characteristics of bone marrow derived mesenchymal stem cells (BM-MSC) from different animal species. Trends Biomater Artif Org, 27: 29-35.

Maiti, S.K. and Singh, G.R. (1996). Transforming growth factor-beta (TGF-β) in bone remodeling, Current Science, 71: 613-617.

Maiti S K, Singh G R. (1998) Bone morphogenetic proteins-novel regulators of bone formation. Indian J Exp Biol, 36: 237-44.

Maiti S K., Ninu, A. R., Sandeep Kumar, Dayamon D. Mathew, Sangeetha, P., Deepika Kritaniya and Naveen Kumar (2013) Mesenchymal stem cells-bioceramic tissue engineered construct for the repair of critical size bone defect in rabbit model. Paper presented in XXXVII Annual Congress of Indian Society for Veterinary Surgery held at Thrissur, Kerala, November 6-8, 2013, page 106.

Maiti SK (2013) Mesenchymal stem cells construct on osteogenesis for repairing large bone defects in animal model, Final Research report submitted to DBT, Govt of India as Principal Investigator.

Maiti, S K and Singh, G. R. (2003) Ceramic biomaterials in reconstructive surgery-A review. Indian J. Vet. Surgery 24: 1-10.

Maiti, S K, Shiva Kumar, M.U., Naveen Kumar, and Ninu, A.R. (2012) Isolation, proliferation And morphological characteristics of Bone-marrow derived Stem Cells (BM-MSC) of different species of animals. 2nd International Conference on Nanobio and Nanosolar conference, Kochi, Kerala, RNM-107, page 114.

Maiti, S K. (1011) Role of mesenchymal stem cell construct on osteogenesis, 35th Annual Conference of ISVS (Kolkata) (Lead Paper) P-168.

Maiti, S K. (2011) Animal Mesenchymal Stem Cells: Isolation, Proliferation, characterization and orthopedic application. 36th World Small Animal Veterinary Congress, Jeju, South Korea. WSAVA Congress Proceeding, SX-P057, page 1143.

Maiti, S K. (2012) Isolation, proliferation and transplantation of bone marrow derived animal mesenchymal stem cells in critical sized bone defects in animal model. Journal of Biotechnology and Biomaterials, 2: 143.

Maiti, S.K., Srivastava L, Shiva Kumar M U and Ninu, A. R. (2012) Isolation, proliferation, in vivo and in vitro application of bone marrow derived mesenchymal stem cells (BM-MSC) in animal model. Proceedings of 4th International Congress on Stem Cells and tissue formation, 18-20th July, 2012, Dresden, Germany, SRD-6, page 105.

Maiti, S K. (2012) Isolation, proliferation and transplantation of bone marrow derived animal mesenchymal stem cells in bone defects in animal model. OMICS 3rd World Congress on Biotechnology, Hyderabad, p-143.

Maiti, S K. (2013) Repair of compact bone critical sized defect with auto, allo and xenogenic mesenchymal stem cells -bioceramic tissue engineered constructs in rabbits" 38th World Small Animal Veterinary Association (WSAVA) Congress, Auckland, New Zealand . Proceeding compendium, page-267.

Maiti, S K. and Spitkovsky, D. (2010) Cultural and morphological characteristics of equine umbilical cord blood and adipose tissue derived mesenchymal stem cells (hrs-UCB-MSC and hrs-AT-MSC). SAPI Silver Jubilee International Conference on Physiological capacity building in livestock under changing climate scenario held at IVRI, Izatnagar. Abstract no-08.3, page 144.

Maiti, S K. and Spitkovsky, D. (2010) Isolation, characterization and proliferation of equine cord blood derived mesenchymal stem cell (hrs-AT-MSC and hrs-UCB-MSC) in different types of serum and oxygen tension environment. 34th Annual Conference of ISVS (Puducherry) Abstract no-SAP-45, P-55.

Maiti, S K., Ninu A R., Remya V., Sivanarayanan T B, Cherian S, Kumar D and Amarpal (2014) Stem cell therapy in animal models of CNS diseases-Therapeutic role, Challenges and Perspectives, Journal of Advanced Veterinary and Animal Research, 1: 75-85.

Maiti, S K., Ninu, A. R., S Gupta, Sandeep Kumar and Naveen Kumar (2012) Characterization of bone marrow derived rabbit mesenchymal stem cells (r-MSC) by flow cytometry and PCR analysis. Proceedings XXXVI Annual Congress of ISVS, Anand, p- 177.

Maiti, S K., Shiva Kumar M U, Ninu, A. R. Sandeep Kumar and Naveen Kumar (2012) In vitro osteogenesis of bone marrow derived rabbit mesenchymal stem cells (r-MSC) Proceedings XXXVI Annual Congress of ISVS, Anand, p- 177.

Maiti S K, Shivakumar M U, Mohan Divya, Kumar N, and Singh KP (2018) Mesenchymal stem cells of different origin-seeded bioceramic construct in regeneration of bone defect in rabbit. Tissue Engineering and Regenerative Medicine 15 (4): 477-492.

Minier K, Toure A, Fusellier M, Fellah B, Bouvy B, Weiss P, Gauthier O. (2014) BMP-2 delivered from a self-cross linkable Ca/P hydrogel construct promotes bone regeneration in a critical-size segmental defect model of non-union in dogs. Vet Comp Orthop Traumatol, 27: 411-21.

Miranville A, Heeschen C, Sengenes C, Curat CA, Busse R, Bouloumie A. (2004) Improvement of postnatal neovascularization by human adipose tissue-derived stem cells. Circulation, 110:349-55.

Mitalipov S, Wolf D (2009) Totipotency, pluripotency and nuclear reprogramming. Adv. Biochem. Eng. Biotechnol, 114: 185–99.

Nadri S, Soleimani M (2007) Isolation murine mesenchymal stem cells by positive selection. *In Vitro* Cell Dev Biol Anim 43: 276-282.

Nair MB, Bernhardt A, Lode A, Heinemann C, Thieme S, *et al.* (2009) A bioactive triphasic ceramic-coated hydroxyapatite promotes proliferation and osteogenic differentiation of human bone marrow stromal cells. J Biomed Mater Res A 90: 533-542.

Nakagami H, Morishita R, Maeda K, *et al.* (2006) Adipose tissue-derived stromal cells as a novel option for regenerative cell therapy. J Atheroscler Throm, 13:77-81.

Neo M, Kotani S, Nakamura T, Yamamuro T, Ohtsuki C, *et al.* (1992) A comparative study of ultra structure of the interfaces between four kinds of surface-active ceramic and bone. J Biomed Mater Res 26: 1419-1432.

Neuss S, Apel C, Buttler P, Denecke B, Dhanasingh A, *et al.* (2008) Assessment of stem cell/ biomaterial combinations for stem cell-based tissue engineering. Biomaterials 29: 302-313.

Niemeyer P, Szalay K, Luginbuhl R, Sudkamp NP, Kasten P. (2010) Transplantation of human mesenchymal stem cells in a non-autogenous setting for bone regeneration in a rabbit critical –size-defect model. Acta Biomaterialia, 6: 900-08.

Niemeyer, P., Thomas Schönberger, Joachim Hahn, Norbert, P. Südkamp, Erich Schneider, Simon Pearce and Stefan Milz. (2008) Xenogenic Transplantation of Human Mesenchymal Stem Cells for Treatment of Critical Size Bone Defects in Sheep. European Cells and Materials 16: 2.

Nilsson, S.K. *et al.*1999 Cells capable of bone production engraft from whole bone marrow transplants in nonablated mice. J. Exp. Med. 189:729-734.

Ninu ,AR, Maiti SK, Palakkara S, Kritaniya D, Mahan T, Kumar N. (2016) In vitro osteoinduction potential of a novel silica coated hydroxyapatite bioscaffold seeded with rabbit mesenchymal stem cell. J Stem Cell Res Therapeutics, 1(2): 49-55.

Ninu AR, Maiti SK, Shiva Kumar MU, Sandeep K, Sangeetha P, Deepika K, Sourabh G, Saxena A and Kumar N (2017) Isolation, proliferation, cherecterization and in vivo osteogenic potential of bone marrow derived mesenchymal stem cells in rabbit model. Indian Journal of Experimental Biology, 55: 79-87.

Owen, M. and Friedenstein, A. J. (1988) Stromal stem cells: marrow-derived osteogenic precursors. Ciba Found Symp., 136:42-60.

Owen, M.E., Cave, J., and Joyner, C.J. (1987) Clonal Analysis in Vitro of Osteogenic Differentiation of Marrow CFU-F. J. Cell Sci., 87: 731–738.

Parker A, Katz A. (2006) Adipose-derived stem cells for the regeneration of damaged tissues. Expert Opin Biol Ther, 6:567-578.

Patel DM, Shah J and Srivastava AS (2013) Therapeutic potential of mesenchymal stem cells in regenerative medicine. Stem Cells International, Article ID: 496218.

Petite, H., Viateau, V., Bensaïd W., Meunier, A., de Pollak, C., Bourguignon, M., Oudina, K. and Sedel, L. (2000) Guillemin G Tissue-engineered bone regeneration. Nature biotechnology 18: 959-63.

Phillips, A.M. (2005) Overview of the fracture healing cascade. Injury, *36*: S5-S7.

Pittenger M F, Mackay A M, Beck S C, Jaiswal R K, Douglas R, Mosca J D, Moorman M A, Simonetti DW, Craig S, and Marshak D R (1999) Multilineage potential of adult human mesenchymal stem cells. Science, 284:143–47

Pluhar GE, Manley PA, Heiner JP, Vanderby R Jr, Seeherman HJ, Markel MD. (2001) The effect of recombinant human bone morphogenetic protein -2 on femoral reconstruction with an intercalary allograft in a dog model. J Orthop Res, 19: 308-17.

Polisetti N, Chaitanya V, Babu PP, Vemuganti GK (2010) Isolation, characterization and differentiation potential of rat bone marrow stromal cells. Neurol India 58: 201-208.

Pontikoglou C, Deschaseaux F, Sensebé L, & Papadaki HA (2011) Bone marrow mesenchymal stem cells: biological properties and their role in hematopoiesis and hematopoietic stem cell transplantation. Stem Cell Reviews and Reports *7*: 569-589.

Prockop, D. J. (1997) Marrow stromal cells as stem cells for nonhematopoietic tissues. Science 276: 71–74.

Rehman J, Traktuev D, Li J, Merfeld-Clauss S, Temm-Grove CJ, Bovenkerk JE, Pell CL, Johnstone BH, Considine RV, MARCh KL. (2004) Secretion of angiogenic and antiapoptotic factors by human adipose stromal cells. Circulation, 16; 109:1292-98.

Remya V, Kumar N, Sharma AK, Sonal, Negi M, Maiti SK, Mathew DD, Shrivastava S and Kurade NP (2014) Acellular fish swim bladder biomaterial construct seeded with mesenchymal stem cells for full thickness skin wound healing in rates. Trends in Biomaterials and Artificial Organs, 28: 1-10.

Salem, H. K. and Thiemermann, C. (2010) Mesenchymal Stromal Cells: Current Understanding and Clinical Status. Stem Cells 28: 585–59674.

Sandeep, K., Maiti, S K., Ansari MM., Naveen Kumar and Asok K Balwada (2014) Effects of medical grade Chitosan powder with xenogenic mesenchymal stem cell for full thickness wound healing in rat model. International Journal of Veterinary Science, 3:129-134.

Sandeep, K., Maiti, S K., Ninu A R., Asok K Balwada, Mathew DD and Kumar, N. (2014) The effects of topical mesenchymal stem cell therapy in full thickness wound healing in a rat model, Trends in Biomaterials and Artificial Organs:28: 65-73.

Sangeetha, P., Maiti, S.K., Singh, K., Gopinathan, A., Kumar, N., Ninu, A.R., Rashmi, Remya V., Sivanarayanan T.B., Tamil Mahan P., Divya Mohan and Mohsina A. (2014) Evaluation of corneal healing with tissue engineered porcine cornea in rabbits. 38th Annual Congress of ISVS, Bikaneer, Compendium, P-218.

Sangeetha, P., Maiti, S.K., Singh, K., Gopinathan, A., Kumar, N., Ninu, A.R., Rashmi, Remya V., Sivanarayanan T.B., Tamil Mahan P., Divya Mohan and Mohsina A. (2014) Evaluation of corneal healing with tissue engineered porcine small intestinal submucosa in rabbits. 38th Annual Congress of ISVS, Bikaneer, P-235.

Sangeetha P. Maiti S K, Divya Mohan, Shivaraju S, Raghuvaran R, Malik Abu Rafee, Bindhuja B V, Naveen Kumar and Raghuvanshi PDS (2017) Mesenchymal stem cells derived from rat bone marrow (rBM MSC): techniques for isolation, expansion and differentiation. Journal of Stem Cell Research & Therapeutics, 3(3): 272-277.

Sangeetha P, Maiti S K, Singh K, Gopinathan A, Singh KP, Mohan Divya, Ninu AR and Kumar N (2017) Evaluation of bio-engineered corneal scaffold for the repair of corneal defect in rabbit model. Indian Journal of Animal Science 87:1332-1339.

Sangeetha P, Maiti S K, Kumar N, Singh K, Gopinathan A, Ninu A R, Remya V, Sivanarayanan TB, Mohsina A, Divya Mohan, Tamilmahan P (2016) Development of bioengineered corneal matrix for reconstruction surgery of eye. Trends in Biomaterials and Artificial Organs: 30 (2): 85-89.

Sangeetha P (2017) Evaluation of Chitosan and Porcine SIS matrix seeded with rat mesenchymal stem cells and m-EGF for the repair of full thickness burn wound in rat model. Ph D thesis submitted to IVRI Deemed University.

Sangeetha P, Maiti S.K, Tamilmahan P, Divya Mohan, Shivaraju S, Raghuvaran R and Naveen Kumar (2018) Evaluation of healing potential of chitosan and porcine small intestinal submucosa seeded with bone marrow derived mesenchymal stem cells for full thickness skin burn wound in rat. 19th Indian Veterinary Congress and Annual Convention of IAAVR, Kolkata, Compendium P: 147-148.

Schöler, Hans R. (2007) "The Potential of Stem Cells: An Inventory". In Nikolaus Knoepffler; Dagmar Schipanski; Stefan Lorenz Sorgner. Humanbiotechnology as Social Challenge. Ashgate Publishing. p. 28.

Sciadini MF, Jojnson KD. (2000) Evaluation of recombinant human bone morphogenetic protein-2 as a bone-graft substitute in a canine segmental defect model. J Orthop Res, 18:289-302

Sekiya I, Larson BL, Smith JR, Pochampally R, Cui JG, *et al.* (2002) Expansion of human adult stem cells from bone marrow stroma: conditions that maximize the yields of early progenitors and evaluate their quality. Stem Cells 20: 530-541.

Shabbir, A., Zisa, D., Leiker, M., Johnston, C., Lin, H., and Lee, T. (2009) Muscular Dystrophy Therapy by Non-Autologous Mesenchymal Stem Cells: Muscle Regeneration without Immunosuppression and Inflammation. Transplantation, 87: 1275–1282.

Shors, E. C. (1999) Coralline bone graft substitutes. Orthop. Clin. North Am., 30: 599.

Strioga M, Viswanathan S, Darinskas A, Slaby O, Michalek J (2012) Same or not the same? Comparison of adipose tissue-derived versus bone marrow-derived mesenchymal stem and stromal cells. Stem Cells Dev 21: 2724-2752.

Tabata, Y. (2003) Tissue regeneration based on growth factor release. Tissue Engineering 9: 5-15

Tae SK, Lee SH, Park JS, IM GI (2006) Mesenchymal stem cells for tissue engineering and regenerative medicine. Biomed Mater 1: 63-71.

Takahashi, K; Yamanaka, S (2006) Induction of pluripotent stem cells from mouse embryonic and adult fibroblast cultures by defined factors. Cell: 126: 663–76.

Takezawa TA (2003) A strategy for the development of tissue engineering scaffolds that regulate cell behavior. Biomaterials, 24: 2267-2275.

Tamilmahan P, Maiti SK, Sangeetha P, Rashmi, Singh P, Divya M and Kumar N. (2016) A combined gene and stem cell therapy for induction of angiogenesis in tissue engineered scaffold for burn wound healing in rat model. 40th Annual Congress of IUSVS, Chennai, Compendium P-176.

Tamilmahan P, Maiti, S K, Sangeetha P, Rashmi, Priya S, Kumar N, Manjunthaachar and Plank C. (2016) Culture, Characterization and differention potential of rat bone marrow derived mesenchymal stem cells. Journal of Stem Cell Research and Therapeutics, 1(5): 193-199

Tokcaer-Keskin Z, Akar A R and Ayaloglu-Butun F (2009) Timing of induction of cardiomyocyte differentiation for in vitro cultured Mesenchymal stem cells: A perspective for emergencies. Can J Physio Pharmacol. 87: 143–50.

Verfaillie C M (2006) "Adult" Stem Cells: Tissue Specific or Not? (Chapter 3). In: "Essential of Stem Cell Biology", (1st Edn), Edited by Robert Lanza, Elsevier Academic Press, P-23.

Vet-Stem Bio Pharma: www.vet-stem.com/technologies: Characteristics of stem cells.

Vidal, M. A., Kilroy, G. E., Johnson, J. R., Lopez, M. J., Moore, R. M. and Gimble, J. M. (2006) Cell growth characteristics and differentiation frequency of adherent equine bone marrow-derived mesenchymal stromal cells: adipogenic and osteogeniccapacity. Vet. Surg. 35: 601–610.

Wang S, Qu X and Zhao RC (2012) Clinical applications of mesenchymal stem cells. J Haematol Oncol, 5:19.

Woodbury D, Schwarz E J and Prockop D J (2000) Adult rat and human bone marrow stromal cells differentiate into neurons. J Neurosci Res, 61: 364-70.

Wu, Y., Chen, L., Scott, P.G. and Tredget, E.E. (2007) Mesenchymal stem cells enhance wound healing through differentiation and angiogenesis. Stem cells 25: 2648-2659.

Yanez R, Lamana ML, Garcia-Castro J, *et al.* (2006) Adipose tissue-derived mesenchymal stem cells have in vivo immunosuppressive properties applicable for the control of the graft-versus-host disease (GVHD). Stem Cells Aug. 24, online version.

Zhu, L., Liu, W., Cui, L. and Cao, Y.L. (2006) Tissue-Engineered Bone Repair of Goat- Femur. Tissue. Eng., 12: 423.

FSC
www.fsc.org
MIX
Papier | Fördert gute Waldnutzung
FSC® C083411

Zeitfracht Medien GmbH
Ferdinand-Jühlke-Straße 7
99095 Erfurt, Deutschland
produktsicherheit@kolibri360.de